M000266550

FASTING FOR HEALTH

And

LONG LIFE

By

HEREWARD CARRINGTON, Ph.D.

(Author of "Vitality, Fasting and Nutrition,"
"The Natural Food of Man," "Death Deferred," etc.)

First Published in 1953
3,000 Impressions

Copyright, 1953,

◆

◆

◆

Printed in the United States of America

Printing Statement:

Due to the very old age and scarcity of this book,
many of the pages may be hard to read due to the
blurring of the original text, possible missing pages,
missing text and other issues beyond our control.

Because this is such an important and rare work, we
believe it is best to reproduce this book regardless of
its original condition.

Thank you for your understanding.

CONTENTS

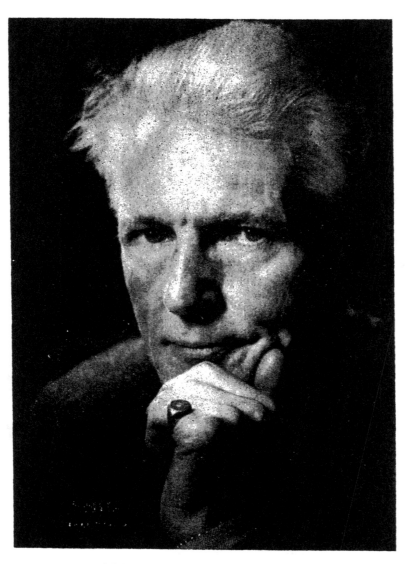

HEREWARD CARRINGTON, Ph. D.

PART I

WHY WE SHOULD FAST WHEN ILL

THE NATURE OF DISEASE

Primitive peoples, as we know, believe that any disease represents the entry into the patient's body of some evil spirit or entity, — which was caused to enter it by some malignant voodoo man or witch-doctor. The unfortunate victim remains so afflicted until he rights a wrong, appeases the witch-doctor, or secures the services of another, whose "magic" is more powerful than that of the original spell-caster. When once this "evil spirit" has been removed, he is well and strong again; if he fails in this, he dies!

Strange as it may seem, a modified form of this same belief underlies public thinking, and constitutes a basic belief of many doctors. True, we no longer believe that an "evil spirit" has entered into the body of a sick person, but it survives in the form of thinking that disease is an "entity" of some sort, which is "caught," and which can be expelled or driven-out by suitable medicines—something in a bottle! When this entity has been expelled, the patient is "cured." Such is the popular conception. . . .

As opposed to this, the Hygienist believes that so-called "diseases" represent merely bodily states or conditions, nearly always self-induced, which are manifested in a series of symptoms, but which are themselves the very processes of cure. As Dr. Emmet Densmore stated, in his book *"How Nature Cures"*:

"Disease and manifestations of disease are friendly efforts and curative actions made by the organism in its efforts to restore the conditions of health. . . The hygienic system teaches that disease is a remedial effort, a struggle of the vital powers to purify the system and recover the normal state. This effort should be aided, directed and regulated, if need be, but never suppressed. . . What is this mysterious thing disease? Simply

3

an effort to remove obstructing material from the organic domain, and to repair damages. Disease is a process of purification. It is a remedial action. It is a vital struggle to overcome obstructions and to keep the channels of the circulation free. . ."

Precisely the same idea was expressed by Miss Florence Nightingale, in her *"Notes on Nursing,"* when she said:

"Shall we begin by taking it as a general principle that all disease, at some period or other of its course, is more or less a *reparative* process, not necessarily accompanied by suffering; an effort of nature to remedy a process of poisoning or decay, which has taken place weeks, months, sometimes years beforehand, unnoticed, — the termination of the disease being then determined?"

So-called disease is, therefore, in the vast majority of cases, merely a *curative effort* on the part of nature; *it is the process of cure itself* — manifested in a set of symptoms. Attempting to "cure" a disease, in the ordinary sense of the word, leads us to a ridiculous paradox: *viz.*, an attempt to cure a curing process! The disease IS the cure. The outward manifestations, the symptoms we notice, represent merely the outward and visible signs of this curative process in action. Any attempt to deal with or smother these symptoms merely retards the process of cure to that extent. Instead of treating symptoms, we should aim at the disease itself, which *causes* them — or rather at the causes of the so-called disease, which are really the dangerous factors involved, and those which have brought about the abnormal conditions noted. Once we have removed these causes, the disease (so-called) disappears, and the symptoms vanish. The patient is then restored to health.

Viewed in this light, everything becomes simple! Toxins and waste material of all kinds accumulate in the body, over a period of weeks, months or years—finally reaching the point when they must be expelled, or deterioration sets in. This violent expulsive effort on the part of nature produces a series of characteristic symptoms. The body attempts in every way possible to expel these poisonous substances — through the bowels, the kidneys, the skin, the lungs, etc. — with the result that these organs are overtaxed and break down under the load. Clogging and toxemia then set in more seriously than ever, and the patient is really ill. Obviously, the only way to relieve this condition is to stop adding to the waste material the body must eliminate, and assist it in every way possible to dispose of what is already there. Once the body is given a chance to "catch up," so to say, and cleanse itself to some extent, the violence of the internal upheaval will subside, and as this becomes more normal, the external symptoms will lessen, and the patient is then said to be "convalescent." If this process continues, he ultimately becomes "cured."

I have used all these terms in a loose sense, because hygienists believe that the so-called "disease" is itself the process of cure, -— as we have seen. What we really mean is that certain causes have been removed, and as they are removed the effects disappear. . . What are these causes, and how are they removed?

The human body is creating certain poisons within itself by the very process of living. If these poisons were not constantly being excreted we should die. Normally, they are disposed of through the various eliminating organs — the bowels, kidneys, skin, etc. If this balance is maintained, the person remains well. If, however, the poisons accumulate more rapidly than they can be disposed of, abnormal conditions develop. These conditions are the so-called "diseases."

Now, it should be obvious that the speediest way to regain health, when this condition develops, is to stimulate the eliminating organs, and at the same time introduce no new poisons into the system. The former is accomplished by means of exercise, bathing, breathing, water-drinking, enemas, etc. But it is highly important to *prevent* the entrance into the body of material which might further clog and block it. This material is our food, and obviously so; for, aside from air and water, this is the *only* material we ever introduce into our bodies, under normal conditions.

The necessity of fasting in times of stress thus becomes evident. Food supplies us with essential nutriment, it is true; but if the body is in no condition properly to utilize this food, it merely decomposes, creates poisons and is pushed through the body without really benefitting it. The thing to do, therefore, is to withhold food, so long as this abnormal state lasts, thereby giving the eliminating organs a chance to dispose of the surplus of material already on hand, and at the same time rest the internal organs, permitting them to accumulate a certain store of vital energy, which would otherwise be expended in the handling and disposal of this extra mass of food-material. The system thus becomes cleansed and purified. It is the simplest and most effective means known to us — and is the course prescribed by nature, when she deprives us, at such times, of our normal appetite.

Practically all diseases thus have a common basis and a common origin. There is a unity and oneness of disease, based on a common denominator. This, in a word, is toxemia. The differing diseases so-called, are but the various means by which nature tries to expel this poisonous material; and the symptoms noted are the outward and visible signs of such curative action. Nature alone cures — whether it be a cut finger, a broken bone or a so-called "disease." All that the doctor can do is to assist nature in this remedial effort. Anything which tends to smother symptoms merely prolongs the effort to that extent. Give nature a chance, and she will heal in every case. A cure will invariably follow — whenever such cure is at all possible.

Most drugs merely subdue pain or smother symptoms. Pain is a warning signal — calling attention to a certain local area which is in dire distress. But this local condition is merely a localized manifestation of a general condition. As Dr. Samuel Dickson remarked: "Properly speaking, there never was a purely local disease." Rectify the general bodily condition, and the local manifestations will disappear. No matter what they may be, or where located, they will vanish when the body as a whole is normal.

Drugs do not *act upon the body;* they are *acted upon by the body.* The action we perceive is the reaction of the body against the drug. It is the effort on the part of nature to expel the poison introduced into the living organism. . . Much the same is true of stimulants. These seem to impart "strength" to the body; but as we know, this is a false strength, denoting merely the waste of the vital energies. If you dig your spur into a tired horse, it will run faster to the corner; but no one thinks that the spur has supplied the horse with fresh energy. It has simply caused the poor animal to expend its reserve energies more quickly. It is the same with stimulants. The false feeling of strength which they impart is fictitious. The same is true of many drugs; *and the same is true of food,* which also acts as a stimulant, giving us a false feeling of strength when a meal is eaten! It is because of this fact that many people feel "weak" when food is withheld.

The simple, basic idea back of the hygienic system is that practically all "diseases," so-called, are but the varied manifestations of a single underlying cause; and that, when this cause is removed, the symptoms automatically vanish. This cause is toxemia and waste material in the body.

All this being so, a single, simple method of treatment should be available. Experience proves to us that such is the case. What is this method? To understand it, we must appreciate the philosophy of the fasting cure. The ground has been laid, and it but remains for us to state the basic principles underlying this method of treatment.

HISTORY OF FASTING

From the very earliest times fasting has been advocated as a curative measure, no less than as a means of attaining higher mystical and spiritual states. It is frequently referred to in the Bible, where "prayer and fasting" were mentioned as joint therapeutic measures. More than two thousand years ago the fasting cure was advocated by the school of the natural philosopher Asclepiades — who also applied the water cure. Even earlier than this, Pythagoras and others instructed their pupils to fast. Plutarch said, "Instead of using medicines, rather fast a day." In an old book, published in the 16th century, entitled *"Of Good Works, and First of Fasting,"* we are told how fasting was used in the primitive church. Throughout the Orient, and among many primitive tribes today, fasting is still an essential part of all magical and psychic initiations.

Christians need hardly be reminded that Christ himself fasted for forty days. . .

It is a great mistake to think of these instances as of only historic interest, or as mere curiosities, representative of the beliefs of uncivilized peoples. Throughout the middle ages many saints and mystics fasted, and, coming to our own times, Doctor Tanner shocked the scientific world when, a little more than half a century ago, he fasted for forty days, and again for forty-two days, on nothing but water. Up to that time, physiologists and medical men generally had repeatedly stated that such a feat would be an impossibility; but Dr. Tanner proved them to be wrong! Since that time, many thousands of persons have fasted for much longer periods of time: both "professional fasters," who placed themselves at the disposal of scientific men, in order that a thorough study might be made of them during this period, and also private individuals, who have cured themselves (often when all other measures had been found to fail) by undergoing long fasts, under the direction of someone with experience in this field of therapy. One of the most famous of these experimental cases was that of Dr. Levanzin, who fasted for 31 days under the auspices of the Carnegie Nutrition Laboratory, of Boston, which institution issued two voluminous reports on fasting and inanition. Dr. Benedict and his associates were astounded at the physical and mental vigor of their patient throughout this experimental period.

Many of the early health reformers advocated fasting as a means of cure: Doctors Graham, Shew, Trall, Oswald, Page, Dodds, and a number of others. Dr. Edward Hooker Dewey became an outstanding figure in this connection, and his writings are classic. Mr. Bernarr Macfadden advocated it from the start, in the pages of *"Physical Culture,"* and was doubtless responsible for spreading the knowledge of the subject throughout the world. Many men and women published books, telling of their own remarkable experiences, and of how they had been "cured," as the result of fasting. My own lengthy book on the subject, *"Vitality, Fasting and Nutrition,"* (of some 700 pages!) was published in 1908. Since then, many other men have taken up the work: Dr. Shelton, who has treated well over twenty thousand cases in this way; Dr. Gian-Cursio, who has treated more than ten thousand cases; Dr. David H. Lipman (of Los Angeles); Dr. Robert G. Wilborn (of Altadena, Calif.); Dr. Gerald Benesh — and many others. This method of treatment is now attracting wider and wider attention and arousing an ever-increasing interest. Slowly but surely the scientific world is being forced to acknowledge the tremendous therapeutic value of fasting, in all cases of sickness, and is applying it more and more in their daily practice. Fasting is at last coming into its own, as a curative measure!

THE PHILOSOPHY OF FASTING

By "the philosophy of fasting" I mean the theory and physiological facts upon which this system of treatment is based. No one should undertake a fast of any length unless he *thoroughly understands* what he is doing and why he is doing it. Moreover he must really "want to fast more than he wants to eat" in order to obtain the maximum benefit from the fast. This he will do if he understands the philosophy underlying it.

I have stressed, over and over again in this book, that the majority of men and women eat too much; the body requires far less food than we think, and can in fact maintain itself in far better health without this constant surfeit. When deprived of food, the body loses approximately a pound a day, and experiments have shown us that this is about the amount we should eat, in order to maintain the body in good condition. Instead of which, most people eat several times this amount — and the wrong kinds of food into the bargain! Is it any wonder that they become ill? The proper amount of food and more than the proper amount cannot possibly have the same effect upon the organism. If one is right the other is wrong. True, Nature has such strong recuperative power that many people can abuse their bodies for years, before they finally break down. But what is the point of doing so, when even these years are filled with troubles and sicknesses of all kinds — as the hundreds of hospitals and thousands of doctors throughout the country amply testify? Something is surely wrong with humanity, in order to render all this necessary; and observations seem to show us that, of all the factors which go to make up this abnormal state of affairs, our erroneous food habits play a predominant role.

When food is eaten over and above the physiological requirements of the body, internal changes begin to occur — things begin to happen. A layer of fatty-tissue is laid down; "colds" are easily "caught"; constipation or diarrhea develop; a lack of energy and "pep" is noted; the individual becomes lazy — and always remember that laziness is a sign of disease! As time passes, other symptoms begin to manifest themselves — slight or grave, as the case may be. Finally the patient breaks down completely and begins to suffer from some acute or chronic "disease." All this because the body has been continuously overloaded and over-worked for a long period of time, in its frantic efforts to dispose of the excess of food material which has been forced into it continuously.

When food is not properly digested, it causes trouble! An excess of protein results in putrefaction; an excess of carbohydrates, in fermentation. Both are bad; both result in unpleasant and ultimately serious symptoms. Gases and poisons are formed within the body, which pass into the blood-stream and affect the tissues and organs, and even the delicate nerve-cells of the brain. The mental and emotional life are affected, no less than the grosser physical elements. Waste material accumulates, toxins are formed, which poison and block the tiny blood vessels. The body becomes choked with the excess. Desperately, nature tries to get rid of this load by driving the eliminating organs to greater and greater efforts, until they break down under the strain. When this occurs, the patient is already in the throes of illness. He is now a really "sick man."

It should be obvious that the thing to do, when such a condition develops, is to give the body a good "house-cleaning" and a rest. The simplest and most effective way of doing this is to put the patient upon a fast. When food is withheld, two things occur: the digestive organs are rested, allowing them to recuperate their energies; and the eliminating organs are given a chance to get rid of the excess of waste material which is clogging the body. As this poisonous matter is removed, the patient recovers.

When the digestive organs are allowed to rest, their vital powers are restored, so that they can handle food adequately, when it is again ingested. All this should be obvious to the merest tyro.

The interesting and amazing thing about a fast is that it attacks and disposes of the *useless* matter *first*

12

— before turning to healthy tissues and organs. One might have thought, a priori, that the reverse of this would be the case; that the healthy reserves of the body would be utilized first of all, and the waste material last. But Nature, in her wisdom, does not proceed in this manner. She carefully preserves the valuable elements in the body — and the more valuable they are the more carefully are they preserved. Waste and poisons are disposed of first; then fatty tissue, and lastly the various organs and tissues of the body, in proportion to their ultimate value to life. In cases of actual *starvation* — when death has resulted — it has been found that the nervous system loses hardly any weight at all! Nature has seen to it that this most precious of our possessions has been imbued with the ability to feed itself at the expense of the rest of the body, and remain practically intact to the very end. (And this, it must be remembered, is in cases of actual starvation — which of course nobody advocates, since, as we shall see, fasting and starvation are two entirely different things: the one being constructive, the other destructive, in their action).

The theory upon which the fasting cure is based lies just here, and I cannot state it more clearly, perhaps, than in the words of Doctor Dewey, when he wrote: "Take away food from a sick man's stomach, and you have begun, not to starve the sick man, but the disease." Or, as Hippocrates put it: "The more you nourish a diseased body, the worse you make it."

Let me quote again the words of Dr. Joel Shew:—

"The principle on which the hunger-cure acts is one on which all physiologists are agreed, and one which is readily explained and understood. We know that in animal bodies the law of nature is for the effete and worn-out and least vitalized matter first to be cast off. . . This then is a beautiful idea in regard to the hunger-cure: that whenever a meal of food is omitted, the body purifies itself thus much from its disease, and it becomes apparent in the subsequent amendment 'both as regards bodily feelings and strength. . .''

We can readily see from the above that, inasmuch as the vital portions of the body are retained relatively intact, during a fast, while the waste material and poisons are eliminated first, a patient is bound to get well long before there is any danger of his "starving to death"; furthermore, that it is impossible for the patient to "starve to death" until the "skeleton condition" is nearly reached — that is, the weight of the bones and viscera. Long before this condition is reached, however, nature will indicate her desire for food — as we shall see, at which time the fast is ready to be broken. Let it be emphasized once again that fasting is *not* starvation, and that no hygienist would recommend the latter, though he might strongly endorse the former. Nearly every 'attack' which has been made upon this method of treatment has been based upon the confusion of these two terms — and of course if you set up a straw man, it is easy to knock him down!

Let it be remembered that "disease, in proportion to its severity, means the loss of digestive conditions and of digestive power." We derive benefit from our food, *not* in proportion to the amount we eat, *but* in proportion to the amount we can properly utilize and assimilate. This fact should ever be kept in mind.

Now, during any diseased condition, food is improperly converted in the body, so that it does not really nourish the patient, but in fact has the effect of starving, poisoning and weakening him at the

14

same time. Remember that the body is only as strong as its weakest link, so that, when it is poisoned and devitalized, every organ and function is devitalized also, and digestion cannot possibly take place normally. It should be obvious that the most sensible thing to do, under these circumstances, is to give the digestive organs a rest, so that they may recuperate their energies, and at the same time permit the various eliminating organs of the body to expel the over-load of toxic material already there.

Inasmuch as the body is essentially *one*, being connected by means of the blood stream, which feeds all parts equally, every part of the body must be benefitted by this means of purification. This enables us to see why it is that seemingly quite unrelated disorders are benefitted by the fast. Probably everyone would be willing to grant that fasting might benefit the digestive organs, because these are most obviously connected with the food we eat; but — until they understand the philosophy of fasting — they cannot see how this procedure could equally benefit such seemingly unrelated conditions as deafness, jaundice, a cold in the head, paralysis, headaches, gastric ulcer; pleurisy, high blood pressure, sinusitis, cough, arthritis, tonsillitis — and scores of other conditions known to "medical science." Yet every one of these so-called diseases is helped or altogether eliminated by means of the fast. Every tissue and organ of the body is reached at the same time and by the same means. No matter what the condition of the patient may be, or the disorder from which he suffers, fasting will benefit him and "cure" the condition with equal certainty and ease. Normal health will be restored in every case — as the records of fasting cases amply testify.

HOW MUCH SHOULD WE EAT?

How much should we eat? We have found that the average fasting patient loses about a pound a day, representing the bodily loss when food is withheld. Clearly, therefore, in order to maintain this balance, about a pound of food should be eaten daily. But, instead of this, we find the average person consuming several times this amount, and this excess of food is only converted and disposed of by imposing an overload upon the digestive and eliminating organs. The vital, recreative powers of the body are so great that a man can over-eat for years before his system finally breaks down; but why impose this excessive labor upon our vital organs if we don't have to? As Dr. T. L. Nichols remarked:

"A man may be able to digest and dispose of three times as much food as he really requires. One ounce more than he requires is a waste of force, a waste of life. We waste life in eating more food than we need, in digesting it, and then in getting rid of it. Here is a triple waste. We have other work to do in this world than eating unnecessary food, and spending our strength for naught."

Or, as Dr. Dewey once said:

"Think of it! Actual soul-power involved in ridding the stomach and bowels of the foul sewage of food in excess, food in a state of decomposition, to be forced through nearly two rods of bowels, and largely at the expense of the soul itself!"

Dr. F. M. Heath again says:

"Thousands there are — yes, millions — who eat more than they can digest, and whose Life Power is so worn-down in the endless struggle with waste food that existence is a hopeless, dragging misery."

Would it not be far simpler, and more rational,

to prevent all this in the first place, by moderate, abstemious living? Instead of eating food in excess, and then becoming ill — and taking pills and laxatives and baths and all the rest, in order to get rid of it — would it not be far easier to eat less in the first place, and thereby obviate the necessity for all these measures — while at the same time maintaining one's self in good health? It would certainly seem so!

REJUVENESCENCE

In many of the lower organisms, it has been proved experimentally that a period of "starvation" actually lengthens life, and produces real rejuvenation. Prof. C. M. Child, of Chicago University, tells us, in his book *Senescence and Rejuvenescence,* that he took some small flat-worms which, when fed, grew old, lazy and infirm, and chopped them up into small pieces, and each piece grew into a new and *young* worm. He took some of the old worms and fasted them for a long time. They grew smaller and smaller, living on their own internal resources for months. Then, when they had been reduced to a minimum size, he fed them. They started to grow and were just as young in physiological condition as they ever were!

The planarian may continue to shrink until reduced to less than one-hundredth of its original size — to a size even below that at which it hatched from the egg. When this point is reached, a supply of food will enable it to grow again.

These reduced worms have the proportions of young, rather than of old worms. They look rejuvenated. Prof. Child alternately fed and starved a group of these worms, and caused them to live over a period of twelve generations. They showed no signs of progressive aging — whenever they were large they were

17

as old as ordinary worms of the same size; whenever they were small they were as young as ordinary young worms. It is stated that "if we choose to go to the trouble we could probably keep a single flat worm alternately going up and down the hill of life and never going beyond a certain age-limit for periods that would make Methuselah seem very short-lived!"

Prof. Child tells us that with abundant food, some species may pass through their whole life-history in three or four weeks, but when growth is prevented, through loss of food, they may continue active and young for at least three years. "Partial starvation inhibits senescence. The starveling if brought back from an advanced age to the beginning of post-embryonic life; it is almost re-born."

These experiments show us very plainly the effects of fasting upon lower organisms; and doubtless some such rejuvenescence is operative in the case of the higher animals — though of course on a lesser scale. We see such effects in many cases of fasting. Youthful vigor is re-established, as many such cases testify.

Let me once again state the case for fasting:—

When a patient is really ill — from any cause whatsoever — the energies of the body are depleted; little power is left for digestion or elimination, and the body is flooded with waste material and poisons of all kinds. The object of fasting is to dispose of these. What possible *use* can food be at such times? Practically no exercise is taken, as a rule, and the patient is often in bed; so there is no breaking-down of tissue on account of exercise. The heat of the body is maintained by the coverings on the bed — in fact, fever is usually present. The energies of the body cannot be replenished by food, even on the current theory of its causation, because the body cannot properly convert and assimilate the food eaten. In fact, experience teaches us that food merely poisons and weakens the body at such times. What possible advantage can there be, therefore, in permitting food? The answer is, None at all! It is a positive detriment, and keeps the patient weak and ill when it is administered. Far better, let nature take its course, and attend to the healing process — as it will, if not interfered with, in any 'diseased' condition, just as it does in the case of a broken bone or the healing of any injury. Nature alone cures! All that anyone can do is to assist her efforts, and permit her to repair the damage. No matter what the condition, or where located, fasting will prove of equal benefit — since it strikes at the real *cause* of the condition; and, when *that* has been eliminated, the resultant effects will automatically disappear.

Fasting, then, is the most logical and the most potent remedial agent known to us, and may be utilized without fear whenever any bodily condition manifests itself indicating a departure from normal health. If it is not a panacea, it comes as near to it as anything well can!

FOOD AND STRENGTH

Perhaps the greatest of all objections to fasting raised by the average person is that the patient would become "so weak," when going without food, that he would be completely incapacitated and bedridden — if he did not actually die during the experiment. This idea that 'we must eat to keep up our strength' is perhaps the most dangerous falsehood ever promulgated, and has been responsible for thousands, if not millions, of deaths. Practically everyone accepts this utterly false notion without question — and doctors have (perhaps unconsciously) been responsible for spreading this untruth, due to their uncritical acceptance of traditional teachings. Yet a few actual experiments and investigations will show it to be entirely untrue.

This idea is doubtless based upon two primary postulates: First, the average person *does* feel depleted and empty, with an "all gone" feeling in the region of his stomach, if he misses one or two meals. From this he draws the conclusion that, if he skipped fifty meals, these feelings would be fifty times as great — in which event he would doubtless be dead from enervation. Besides, most people love to eat, and it's hard to get them to resist food!

The second is the teaching of accepted physiology — that the bodily energies are directly dependent upon the food we eat. Into this we shall enter in some detail immediately.

It must be understood, first of all, that the seeming weakness and "all gone" feeling which we experience, when missing a meal, is due primarily to two factors, and not to the actual lack of food. These are (1) the loss of stimulation — physical and mental — which food ordinarily affords. *Food is a stimulant* — particularly if it is hot food of the ordinary kind. The sudden withdrawing of this stimulus is noted in a certain reaction. When the chronic alcoholic suddenly stops drinking, a similar 'let-down' is noted. But this would not be because the system is being deprived of nutriment, but because the customary stimulation is suddenly withdrawn. Much the same is true of food. (The mental factor is also highly important here.)

(2) During the first day or two of a fast, the patient is apt to become hungry at every meal time,

20

due to what is known as "habit hunger." A gnawing sensation will be experienced in the stomach, accompanied by a feeling of emptiness. If a glass of water is drunk, and the mind immediately distracted to other things, this will pass off, and will not be experienced again until the next regular meal time. After the first two or three days, this will not as a rule be experienced again. Hunger will disappear, and will not return again until the fast is ready to be broken — whenever that may be. Nature will always set this time-limit, and the return of natural hunger will indicate that the fast is terminated and the body again ready for food.

As the fast progresses, the strength of the patient will be found to increase — especially if he is seriously ill at the beginning of the fast. As the elimination of toxins proceeds, the energy of the body will be found to return. I have known patients who were so weak, at the beginning of the fast, that they could scarcely walk down stairs, but who, after twenty or more days on nothing but water, were walking four and five miles a day! If our strength depended upon food, in the sense usually supposed, this would be a paradox indeed!

Once the philosophy of fasting be understood, however, all this is at once understood and readily explained. It is no paradox at all, but precisely what we should expect. The truth of the matter is this: Weakness is due to *disease,* not to lack of food. As the body is cleansed, so does strength return. Rid the body of toxins — the true cause of disease (so-called) — and energy will flow freely through the body, revitalizing it and imparting to it a sense of added vitality. A really ill person will feel better and stronger as the fast progresses.

Remember, always, that we normally derive bene-

21

fit from our food *not* in proportion to the amount we eat, but in proportion to the amount we can properly utilize and assimilate. In most cases of illness, this amount is virtually *nil*. The digestive organs are over-worked and their available energies at a low ebb, due to the tax which has been constantly imposed upon them. The digestive juices are vitiated and scanty; the whole system is choked and blocked with an excess of waste material. Under these circumstances, none of the food is properly converted, but is sluggishly pushed through the intestinal tract in a state of semi-decomposition. The various eliminating organs, already over-worked, cannot handle and dispose of this new load, with the result that it accumulates, forms excess fat and, later, acids and toxins of all kinds. The very surfeit of food prevents any of it from being properly digested, with the result that the patient is starved and poisoned at the same time. The only logical course to pursue, under the circumstances, is to give the system a chance to catch-up and eliminate this excess; and when it has done so, the food will once more be properly converted and utilized, and we will derive the benefit from it in the form of wholesome nourishment. Fasting is the most rapid and effective way to accomplish this result.

With the disposal of this waste material, and its accompanying toxins, strength returns. Remember that poison is the great devitalizer, and the degree of our bodily energies depends upon the cleanliness of the organism. The healthier the body, the more energy it possesses. That is why athletes go into training; it is a matter of common observation. The man whose tissues are physiologically clean, who "hasn't an ounce of fat on him," is the man who is well and fit, and capable of great exertion. Knowing this, how can people be so silly as to keep stuffing themselves with food, when they take no exercise, and are already weakened and devitalized by the excess of food they have already eaten?

It is the greatest mistake in the world to 'tempt the appetite' of the sick person, and induce him to eat 'just a little something,' when his natural aversion to food clearly indicates that his body neither needs nor craves it. Nature is calling for a fast; and the sicker the individual the more necessary the fast becomes. When deprived of food, the body lives on its own reserves, and it can do so for days and weeks, with only added benefit, when the body is already over-burdened with an excess of food material. It should be permitted to dispose of what is already there, before new supplies of food are added.

If we observed animals (even our domestic animals, whose habits have been largely perverted) we should notice that they invariably refuse to eat, when ill or indisposed. A dog or a cat will refuse food at such times, drinking a little water, but disdaining all solid food. Instinct tells them to fast, and they do. Dr. Oswald had a dog that fell out of a second story of a barn, and broke several ribs and injured itself internally, as the result of the fall. This dog refused all solid food for twenty-six days, getting out of its bed on the twenty-seventh day, as lively and active as ever. If only human beings were as wise as that, what an amount of suffering humanity would spare itself!

Unfortunately, the average person is so wedded to his food, and so hypnotized by the belief that he will immediately collapse if he is deprived of it, that the very last thing he consents to do is to undertake a fast. It is for this reason that the majority of fasting cases are those that have tried everything else, without relief, and only come to this as a last resort. It is the "last straw" at which they clutch frantically, in their effort to preserve life. If only they had undertaken a fast weeks or perhaps years before, they would have been spared all those intervening months of suffering; and further, the necessitated fast would then have been much shorter and easier, since far less time would have been necessitated in bringing about normal conditions. The omission of a few meals now and then would obviate the necessity of such long fasts, since this simple procedure would keep them in good condition and a state of normal physiological balance.

As before stated, this idea that strength depends upon our food, and that we become weak in its absence, is based upon current physiological teachings, which directly or indirectly emphasize this point. The orthodox scientific theory, briefly stated, is approximately as follows:

Consider an ordinary steam engine. A certain amount of fuel is shovelled into the engine and burnt up. Heat and energy are evolved in consequence. There is an invariable equivalence between the amount of fuel suppied and the work done. The more fuel consumed, the greater amount of heat and energy released. This relationship can be established mathematically.

The human body is said to resemble the steam engine. The fuel is the food, while the energy furnished by its consumption heats the body and supplies its energy. The wastes of the tissues of the body are, of course, replaced by the food-material itself.

This is the analogy given us in all text books on physiology. Upon it is based the idea that food gives us "strength," and that we become "weak" when deprived of food. And yet even a little reflection would serve to show us the falsity of this analogy, and show us that the body does not resemble a steam engine, in the sense ordinarily implied. This may be proved in two or three ways.

In the first place, it should be obvious to us that, at the end of the day, when we are tired as the result of our labors, and our energies are low, we seek rest and sleep, in order to replenish them. This fact alone differentiates the human body from the steam engine. Nothing but sleep will restore our energies — as we realize from experience. Were the common mechanical analogy true, we should merely have to eat more food, and then burn it up by exercise, deep breathing, etc., in order to restore our energies, — whereas we know that this is not the case. Protoplasm must be rested, and the unique recuperative power of sleep is well known. There is reason to believe that many mysterious vital processes go on in sleep, of a nature wholly unknown to present-day science. Be that as it may, the fact remains that sleep and only sleep restores our vital powers, and that a person can live much longer without food than he can without sleep. The steam engine does not need to sleep, whereas the human body does. This fact alone should prove to us the difference between them, and the obvious falsity of the analogy which is usually drawn, in an attempt to prove that these two "machines" closely resemble one another.

What seems to happen is that the nervous system, and the body generally, is somehow re-charged, during the hours of sleep, by some cosmic energy, which flows into the body at such times. A closer analogy, perhaps, would be that of the electric motor, which is similarly recharged, or the electric battery. Work is done only when this accumulated energy is being spent or discharged. Never forget that energy is invariably noted by us, *as* energy, only in its expenditure, never in its accumulation! If sleep and only sleep can thus 'recharge' us, the old analogy of the steam engine breaks down, and is shown to be inapplicable to the human body.

Another fact which we must keep constantly in mind is that, in fasting cases, the energy of the body is frequently seen to increase, as the days pass; whereas, if the old analogy were true, we should get weaker and weaker when food (the source of our energy) is withheld. Yet the facts prove the contrary — as anyone conversant with fasting cases will testify. It is true that the reserves of the body are drawn upon, at such times, and consumed during the fasting period. But if this potential food-reserve is constantly there, as it obviously is, why worry about the omission of a few meals, and why the contention that a huge daily intake of food is necessary, in order to "keep up the strength," when by their own admission this lasting reserve is there? The argument obviously does not hang together.

The function of food, therefore, is to supply the tissues and organs of the body with the pabulum they need (when this food can be profitably utilized) and the bodily heat [1]; but not the energy of the body, which is replaced by rest and sleep. Were this theory true, it would at once show us the fallacy of the argument that strength depends directly upon food, and that we become weak immediately when it is with-

[1] Even this may be questioned—at least in the *direct* sense ordinarily supposed. In my *Vitality, Fasting and Nutrition*, I devoted some eighteen pages to a discussion of this question. See "Body Temperature."

held. Fasting cases prove the contrary.

The vital energy plays-upon and functions *through* the body. The latter is the mechanism for its expression. It does not manufacture energy, it transmits it. Years ago, Professor William James wrote a little book entitled *Human Immortality,* in which he advanced the theory that the human brain, instead of being a thought-*creating* machine, may be a thought-*transmitting* machine; and that the relation between mind and brain might be in the nature of a 'transmissive function.' The same analogy might be applied to the *whole* of the bodily energies. On this view, the amount of energy transmitted would be proportional to the degree of cleanliness of the body, and its "polarity," and to nothing else. As Professor F. C. S. Schiller expressed it:

"If the material encasement be coarse and simple, as in the lower organisms, it permits only a little intelligence to permeate through it; if it is delicate and complex, it leaves more pores and exits, as it were, for the manifestations of consciousness."

One has only to extend this idea to the *whole* of the vital energies, instead of to the mental energies alone, to see its reasonableness and applicability. If the body is clean, and in a state of health, an abundance of vital energy flows through it. If, on the other hand, it is choked and blocked by waste material, and poisoned by toxins, but little energy can be manifested. And this is precisely what we observe in all diseased conditions. Then, as we know, the energies are at a low ebb, and only return as health is restored. Inasmuch as fasting is the most rapid and effective way of bringing this about, it follows that the energies will return as the channel for their manifestation becomes cleansed. The fact of the matter is that food, during any illness, — instead of giving us strength, — keeps us weak and devitalized; and the withholding of food will increase our energies by permitting them to function. This is one of the main results accomplished by fasting. [2]

THE NO-BREAKFAST PLAN

"Woe unto thee, O land, when thy king is a child, and thy prince eat in the morning!

"Blessed art thou, O land, when thy king is the son of nobles, and thy princes eat in due season, for strength, and not for drunkenness!"

—*Ecclesiastes*, X, 16-17.

The no-breakfast plan is a term first propounded by Dr. Dewey, and the idea was strongely advocated by him. He advised many of his patients to omit breakfast altogether, taking only a glass of water, and go until the mid-day meal before partaking of solid nourishment. The benefits which many of his patients derived from this simple procedure were extraordinary. They rid themselves of many minor ills, and doubtless rendered a long fast unnecessary, — which might otherwise have been necessitated.

The principles upon which the 'no-breakfast plan' rested were mainly two: it reduced the total quantity of food eaten during the day; and, second, inasmuch as the main function of food is to replace broken-down tissue, this waited upon exercise to produce this result, before supplying the body with food necessary to replace the waste.

As Dr. Dewey remarked:—

". . . There is no natural hunger in the morning

(2) In the light of the above theory, new light is thrown upon the nature of sleep, death, and many other psycho-biological problems, as I pointed out in my former book upon this subject: *Vitality, Fasting and Nutrition.* The reader is referred to it for further discussion of these questions.

after a night of restful sleep, because there has been no such degree of cell-destruction as to create a demand for food at the ordinary hour of the American breakfast. Sleep is not a hunger-causing process.''

Eating a hearty breakfast is merely making a bread-basket of your stomach, in anticipation of the time when this food will be needed. The cart has in fact been placed before the horse. Instead of first creating a desire for food, — by exercise and general work, — and then supplying this demand, according to the dictates of normal hunger, the food is supplied first, and the exercise taken later! In short, hunger should be *earned*, before it is appeased; and the postponement of breakfast creates this healthy appetite — which will make itself manifest when the system really begins to crave food.

It is true that many people find breakfast the hardest meal in the day to omit. Those who have been accustomed to eat a 'hearty' breakfast, should begin by tapering-off the amount of food, cutting it down as the days pass until only a minimum is eaten. It is not necessary to omit breakfast altogether, if the other meals are light and due care is taken with the diet; moreover, as Dr. Dewey said, it is not necessary to go until twelve or one o'clock before eating a snack of some sort — assuming of course that the patient is not on a fast, and is living a normal life. But it is undoubtedly true that a minimum breakfast makes for efficiency — no matter what the 'vitamin experts' may contend. Large numbers of people are finding this out for themselves, and admit that they feel much better as the result of omitting or greatly reducing the early meal. It is the *stimulation* of the morning food, plus coffee, as a rule, which is missed, rather than the food itself. On a simple, bland diet this stimulating

29

quality of food is always reduced to a minimum, and a fast, or any radical alteration in the diet, made much easier because of this.

PROS AND CONS OF FASTING

Summing-up the *pros* and *cons* of fasting as a therapeutic measure, Doctor Herbert M. Shelton (who, be it remembered, has treated many thousands of patients by these means) has this to say:—

Fasting does not cause the stomach to 'shrink up.'

Fasting does not cause the walls of the stomach to grow together.

Fasting does not cause the digestive fluids of the stomach to turn upon it and digest the stomach.

Fasting does not paralyze the bowels.

Fasting does not impoverish the blood nor produce anemia.

Fasting does not produce acidosis.

Fasting does not cause the heart to weaken or collapse.

Fasting does not produce malnutritional edema.

Fasting does not produce tuberculosis nor predispose to its development.

Fasting does not "reduce resistance" to "disease."

Fasting does not injure the teeth.

Fasting does not injure the nervous system.

Fasting does not injure any of the vital organs.

Fasting does not injure the body's glands.

Fasting does not cause abnormal psychism.

Turning to the positive side of the picture, fasting insures the following benefits:

(1)   It gives the vital organs a complete rest.

(2)   It stops the intake of food, which may decompose in the intestines and poison the body.

(3)   It empties the digestive tract and disposes of putrefactive bacteria.

(4)   It gives the organs of elimination an opportunity to catch-up with their work, and promotes elimination.

(5)   It re-establishes normal physiological chemistry and normal secretions.

(6)   It promotes the breaking-down and absorption of exudates, deposits, 'diseased' tissues, and abnormal growths.

(7)   It restores a youthful condition to the cells and tissues, and rejuvenates the body.

(8)   It permits the conservation and re-canalization of energy.

(9)   It increases the powers of digestion and assimilation.

(10)   It clears and strengthens the mind.

(11)   It improves function throughout the body.

What more could be asked of any system of therapy?

PART II

CASE-HISTORIES

CASE-HISTORIES OF FASTING PATIENTS

Since the beginning of the present century — when therapeutic fasting was first called to public attention by Doctors Tanner and Dewey — many thousands of patients have been treated by this method, or have voluntarily undergone fasts themselves. The number of cases treated by Dr. Dewey is unknown, but they must have been many; and, since then, specialists in this field have supervised hundreds upon hundreds of such cases: e.g., Doctor Shelton, well over twenty thousand, Doctor Gian-Cursio more than ten thousand, while Doctors Rabagliati, Page, Oswald, Shew, Lipman, Lackey, Wilborn, Benesh, Trall, Macfadden, and many others — including the present writer — have likewise observed hundreds of fasting cases. Many men — such as J. Austin Shaw, Upton Sinclair, Dr. I. J. Eales, Van R. Wilcox, etc. — have written books about their own fasts, while an enormous literature has grown up about the subject. Even "orthodox" medical Journals have given it serious consideration, and physiologists have made extended studies of patients undergoing a prolonged period of "inanitian." There is really no longer any valid excuse for the present woeful ignorance on the part of the public as to the validity of this method of treatment, but such nevertheless seems to be the case, and it is in the hope of dispelling some of this ignorance that the present little book has been written — attempting to present, in concise and popular form, the basic principles upon which this system rests.

It must be understood that, in the cases which follow, the fast was undertaken for the sole purpose of curing the patient of some "disease." They were not "experimental" fasts, nor were they cases of "starvation." They are representative cases of thera-

35

peutic fasting. Scores — hundreds — of such cases could be given, but space must limit me to a few illustrative instances. They will perhaps suffice to bring home the potency of this method of treatment.

George E. Davis, age 61, fasted to fifty days. Entire right side paralyzed; mental depression, constant drowsiness, mentality impaired, speech impeded. Weight at commencement of fast, 228 lbs. Stomach girth, 45 inches. Weight at close of fast, 174 lbs.; girth, 38½ inches. Some six weeks after breaking the fast, his weight was 184 lbs; his girth 39 inches. Mr. Davis wrote:

"I am cured of paralysis. My mentality is clear and normal; my entire digestive system is apparently perfect; my vision is better than for years; my hand and arm are strong; I have no dread of a second stroke; I have no sleepy spells; I feel lighter all over; and when I am weary I am quite refreshed and ready for further exertion after a short rest, which is always — as is my food — simply delicious. I feel much younger, and my neighbors say I 'look it.' "

Some months later, Mr. Davis wrote that he was still in excellent health and spirits.

Mrs. I. Matthews, age 45, fasted for twenty-two days. Weight at commencement, 150 pounds; at conclusion, 123 pounds. Chronic catarrh and frequent 'colds.' Completely rid of her catarrh, and did not have a cold for months following the fast.

Rev. N. J. Lohre, age 35, fasted for ten days. Lost 13 pounds. Had suffered for several years from alternating constipation and diarrhoea, with headaches and insomnia. Condition completely rectified by fasting; no return of former distressing symptoms.

Professor F. W., age 46, fasted for twenty days. Lost 24 pounds during this period. Incipient diabetes.

Examination at the conclusion of the fast showed that symptoms had entirely disappeared. Sugar content of urine normal, as reported by two laboratories.

George W. Tuthill, age 47, fasted 41 days. Weight at the conclusion of the fast, 98 pounds; skeleton condition nearly reached. Partial paralysis; constant headaches; hearing and vision impaired. The patient had been suffering for more than ten years, during which period he had experimented with "treatments" of every kind. *Within ten days* the patient's paralysis had almost entirely disappeared, and he was enabled to walk about, as he did until the end of the fast. Headaches vanished; hearing and vision almost normal at its conclusion. Patient remained in active health until I lost track of him, when he moved to another city, some weeks later.

Mrs. J. F. C., age 47, mother of five children. Fasted for 28 days. Weight at beginning, 127 pounds; at end, 103 pounds — a loss of 24 pounds. Severe bronchial trouble, attended by constant coughing. Had been under treatment for more than six years, with no benefit. After only a few days' fast, the soreness left the throat and chest, and quantities of phlegm were coughed-up. The patient continued to improve, feeling better and stronger as the fast progressed. On the 28th day, natural hunger terminated the fast, though the patient remained on liquid food for six days longer. None of former symptoms in evidence. Patient remained well and strong, and in excellent spirits.

Mrs. T. A., age 50, fasted 34 days, for indigestion and severe liver trouble. Weight 117 pounds; fell to 92 pounds at conclusion of the fast. Her illness had extended over a period of thirty years. Headaches and liver trouble completely disappeared and patient continued to enjoy better health than she had for years past.

Robert B., age 29 years; fasted for 17 days, for deafness and chronic catarrh. Weight 135 pounds; fell to 118 pounds. Patient totally blind. Hearing grew much worse for several days; then a quantity of pus was discharged and patient felt great relief. He could now hear better than he had in years. He had been pronounced incurably deaf, but at the end of the fast he could hear sounds several feet away. The fast was unfortunately broken prematurely, owing to the fact that the patient had to return home (another city) by a certain date. When last seen, the patient was feeling well and strong, and greatly encouraged by the results of his fast. He stated that he intended to take another one later. (Whether he did so or not could not be verified).

Miss Louise W. Kops, age 27, fasted for 16 days. Weight at commencement, 128 pounds; at conclusion, 117 ¼ pounds. Headaches; pains in back and side, and general feeling of depression. Walked and attended to regular business (as a visiting nurse) throughout the fast. Felt well and strong; urine became clear. Temperature approximately normal throughout the fast. Walked one-and-a-half miles on last day; ended by "feeling very well."

J. Austin Shaw, age 55; fasted for 45 days, during which time he lost 25 pounds. Mental and physical powers impaired; eye-sight affected. Health and strength increased daily as fast progressed, and patient worked from twelve to eighteen hours a day throughout the entire period. The patient kept a diary, the last entry being: "If anything, I find my strength greater this morning than on any of the forty-five days, which close at six tonight. . . ." Mr. Shaw subsequently published the details of his fast in his book, *The Greatest Thing in the World.*

Diana Young, fasted in 1939 for 42 days — the last ten days, however, on diluted fruit juices. Weight at commencement of fast, 115 pounds; at end, 85 pounds. Gall stones, ulcerated teeth and badly ingrowing toe-nails. Both teeth and toe-nails had to be operated upon immediately, according to the best "authorities." Needless to say, the gall stones also necessitated an immediate operation!

This was one of those rare cases where the patient felt hungry almost constantly throughout the fast — after the first few days. She now is inclined to think this was mostly psychological. Took enemas and irrigations daily. Felt weak, suffered from headaches, lassitude, and pains in the legs, arms and back. On the sixteenth day, the stones were passed, and patient then felt much better. Continued to fast despite unpleasant symptoms, and 'good' and 'bad' days fluctuated. Patient slept well almost throughout.

X-rays taken soon after the conclusion of the fast showed no abscesses, and she still has her teeth, which are sound and well. Ingrowing toe-nails also cured, so that no operation was necessitated, and she still has them, in good condition. Felt exceedingly well after the fast, and has had no trouble since!

Mrs. A. E. R., age 69 years, fasted (not completely, since she took fruit juices, etc.) for three weeks, during which period she lost more than forty pounds — doubtless due to her excessive weight, as she weighed 225 pounds at its commencement. The patient was excessively active, being on her feet and moving about constantly. Had suffered for more than thirty years from chronic colds, diarrhoea, rigidity of the knee joints, varicose veins, etc. During that time she had been treated by many well-known physicians, to no avail. During her three weeks' fast, all former symptoms entirely disappeared, including the varicose veins, so that the elastic stockings, which she had worn for years, were discarded. Headaches, colds, diarrhoea and other troubles entirely eliminated.

Mrs. R. T., age 32, fasted for 18 days. Weight at beginning of fast, 98 pounds! Had suffered for several years from headaches, nausea, loss of appetite, and severe pain in the ascending colon. All symptoms disappeared during the fast, except that a slight pain still persisted in right side. After breaking the fast, the patient went on an abstemious diet, limited to two small meals a day. She gained weight and strength daily, and at the end of three months the pain in the side had completely disappeared. No recurrence. . . . Whatever the cause of the pain — whether a growth or not — it had evidently been removed by the fasting and her subsequent abstemious life.

G. W. S., age 45, completely bedridden for more than nine years; paralysis of the entire body, with anaesthesia. Many forms of treatment had been tried, in vain. At the conclusion of the fast, the patient could sit up in bed, and move both arms and legs slightly, and also his fingers and toes. A complete cure was not of course effected in this case. But the interesting fact connected with it was that the patient fasted for the extraordinary length of time of *seventy-nine days* — with added strength and improvement! What reply would be made to this by those objectors who contend that they "get so weak" when they skip an occasional meal?

C. G. Patterson, age 69½ years, fasted for 31 days. Weight at conclusion of fast, 102¾ pounds. Patient had been treated for seventeen years, with no improvement in his condition. Mr. Patterson kept a Diary throughout the fast, from which I quote the following:

August 9th: "At this moment I could not define any particular change in my physical condition since the fast began five days ago.

August 15th: "For the first time since beginning this fast I perceived that the nauseating smell so long characterizing my urine has considerably lessened; it is now of a natural color, clear and almost odorless.

August 19th: "I have noticed recently that, instead of proverbially cold feet, I have warm ones now; they are never uncomfortable of late.

August 20th: "Within a few days I have observed that my finger nails have grown very much harder than usual. . . .

August 22nd: "I find, since beginning this fast, that my nerves have improved immensely. I can now write with a steady, confident hand; this has not been the case before in several years.

August 30th: "There has been no loss of strength today; on the contrary, I think I feel rather more aggressive than for some time past.

September 2nd: "My strength remains without perceptible change, and I have no craving for food. . ."

The patient broke his fast the next day, and some time later he was enabled to write:

"My weight has increased from 102 ¾ pounds, on Sept. 3rd, to 114 pounds today. My skin has a healthy glow; my vision is certainly clearer; my ability to endure physical exercise is greater than for several years past, and, generally, my health is good. . . . My hands and feet are now the same temperature as the rest of my body."

Doctor I. J. Eales, fasted for 30 days, during

which time he lost 28 pounds. Acute albuminuria, functional disorder of the heart, excess weight. Dr. Eales made a detailed study of his own case, which was reported in the *"St. Louis Republic,"* June 30, 1907. (See my *Vitality, Fasting and Nutrition,* pp. 216-20, for a full account of this case). All symptoms entirely disappeared, and Doctor Eales was enabled to write:

".... I have disproved some of the theories taught for years in some of our standard text books. I have tested my strength and endurance almost daily, and at the end of a thirty-day fast I was able to lift and hold a man of 250 pounds weight by grasping him under the arms. . . ."

Van R. Wilcox, fasted for 60 days — as fully described in his own little book *Correct Living.* Suffered from boils, eczema, hemorrhoids, partial paralysis, defective eyesight, baldness, rheumatism, kidney disease, constipation alternating with diarrhoea, etc. Mr. Wilcox was completely cured of every one of his many ailments. . . . In so fine a physical condition was he, indeed, that he undertook a walk from New York to San Francisco, which he completed in 167 days. He accomplished this feat on two small meals a day, never once eating breakfast. Many times he ate nothing for one or two days at a time. Boils, pimples, skin eruption, etc., entirely disappeared, and his weight increased from 105 to 160 pounds. Mr. Wilcox tells the whole story in his book, above mentioned.

The following cases were sent me by Dr. Herbert M. Shelton, as recently observed by him:—

Single woman, age 27, goitre, two years, nervous symptoms; condition had grown steadily worse under two years of medical care. Fast of 28 days resulted in disappearance of all thyroid enlargement and all nervous symptoms. No recurrence of symptoms after one year.

Married woman, age 36, asthma for two years. Usual medical care proved unavailing. Fast of twenty-five days resulted in disappearance of all asthmatic symptoms. Patient returned to Canada and indulged in winter sports. No recurrence of symptoms after a year.

Married woman, age 37, migraine for over fifteen years. Continued use of pain-killing drugs had converted her into a dope-addict. Forty days of fasting were accompanied by severe headache, much vomiting of bile and occasional spasticity of hands and feet. Complete recovery resulted only after three subsequent fasts of three to four days each.

Married man, age 46, one kidney removed, large stone in other kidney. After twelve days of fasting, stone crumbled and began to pass piece by piece. In addition to large amounts of small pieces of stone that caused no pain, no less than twenty pieces large enough to cause much pain were passed during the next fourteen days of fasting. Patient recovered.

Man, age 43, barber, paralyzed on whole of right side. Medical prognosis. incurable. An uneventful fast of twenty-eight days restored full use of arm and lower limb, so that patient returned to his work as a barber.

Widow woman, age 38, dentist. Arthritis of right arm, shoulder and upper spine for three years. Usual medical care registered the usual failure. Fast of twenty-five days resulted in disappearance of all pain and inflammation, normal movement to all joints and partial reduction of enlarged finger joints — *Heberden's Notes.*

Married woman, age 28, nurse. Seventy pounds

overweight. Underwent a twenty-five day fast for reducing, regained sight in eye that had been totally blind for over ten years. No recurrence of blindness after eight years.

Married woman, age 48, housewife, neuritis of right arm. Had a fast of 36 days. Regained hearing in right ear, which had been deaf for twenty-five years.

Dr. David H. Lipman (Chiropractor) — of Los Angeles — has treated many cases by fasting, some of them extending over periods of fifty days and longer. To mention briefly a few of these, extracted from his case-histories, which he kindly lent me:

Case 371: Woman, age 65, fasted for 48 days. Weight at conclusion of fast 106 pounds. Pulse 60; Temp. 97°. (on last day of fast). Patient felt extremely well and full of energy at end.

Case 245: Woman, 35 years; fasted for 26 days, down to weight of 91 pounds. Had suffered for many years from gas, constipation, cold hands and feet, chronic 'tired feeling' . . . Bowel movements and large amounts of gas throughout fast. At conclusion, urine clear, eyesight greatly improved; 'felt like a new-born person.' Pulse 80. Her Diary stated that she "felt so strong it seemed I had not fasted at all." All former trouble removed; no more tired feeling.

Case 152: Man, age 23, fasted for 22 days, for enlarged thyroid, skin eruptions, rapid pulse, chronic constipation. Had suffered for ten years. Skin completely cleared. Pulse at beginning of fast, 84; at conclusion, 60. Temp. 97° F. Felt well and strong.

Case 86: Woman, age 47, fasted for 33 days; for chronic headaches, constant cough, other complications. Pulse at end of fast, 60; Temp. 98.6° F. Stated that she felt "fine" at conclusion.

Case 178: Woman, age 65; fasted 14 days, for varicose veins, poor circulation, bad breath, catarrh. Pulse and temperature normal at conclusion. Varicose veins almost completely gone.

Case 203: Man, fasted 22 days, for spastic colon, piles, skin eruption. All these conditions cleared up. Weight at end, 132 pounds. Felt better than he had in years.

In his book, *The No Breakfast Plan*, Doctor Dewey refers to the following cases, among others:

C. C. H. Cowen—catarrh; fasted forty-two days.

Milton Rathbun—Obesity; twenty-eight days.

Milton Rathbun—(second fast) thirty-six days.

Estella Kuenzel — Mental disorder; forty-five days.

Leonard Thress—Dropsy; fifty days.

Elizabeth Westing—forty days.

Rev. C. H. Dalrymple—forty days.

Many similar cases may be found in the literature of fasting, covering periods up to fifty days and more — for a great variety of ills. The majority of such cases had tried everything else in vain, only undertaking a fast as a 'last resort'! All advocates of fasting well know that such is usually the case!

(See Appendix I. for additional cases.)

PART III

SPECIAL POINTS OF INTEREST

HOW LONG SHOULD ONE FAST?

Generally speaking, it is a mistake to set a time-limit on the length of the fasting period. One cannot say beforehand, "I intend to fast for ten days," — or whatever length of time he may have in mind. His body may have other views! It may be that this man requires only a three-day fast, or he may require one or twenty days — or longer. It all depends on his condition at the time. Nature will always indicate when the fast is terminated and ready to be broken — by the return of natural hunger, and by various symptoms which are described elsewhere. . . . If a man requires a fifteen day fast, and he breaks it at the end of ten days, merely because he has set an arbitrary time-limit to his fast, he has broken it prematurely, and he will fail to derive the benefits from the fast which he would have, had he permitted it to continue. In fact, he may run into a set of unpleasant reactions. On the other hand, it is most unwise to continue the fast, once nature has signalled its termination, merely because he has made up his mind to fast so-many days. Either method is harmful. The only logical procedure is to fast until nature indicates her desire for food (as she invariably will) and then and then only should the fast be broken.

The best way is to go along from day to day, noting symptoms, but otherwise disregarding the body and paying no particular attention to it. Fast as long, but only as long, as may be necessary. Nature, and not the patient, will dictate how long this should be.

WHAT IS THE BEST TIME
TO TAKE A FAST?

All fasting patients tend to feel cold, as the days pass, and they should be kept warm — either by putting them to bed or by plenty of heavy clothing if they go out. For this reason, summer is usually a better time to take a fast than winter; it is somewhat easier on the patient. However, it may be taken at any time of the year, and equal benefits are derived from it, no matter when it is undertaken. If the patient is really ill, then of course the fast must be started immediately, whatever the temperature may be. If he waited for the summer to come 'round, he might be dead in the meantime — and he wouldn't want that! On general principles, summer is easier than winter, but it is really immaterial when the fast may be undertaken.

Some people, it is true, rarely feel the cold at all, and can tramp 'round in the ice and snow with perfect comfort. But they are the exceptions. It is far better to be on the safe side, and see to it that your patient is warm and relaxed while fasting. If *you* are the subject, the same of course applies to yourself!

CAN'T I EAT "A LITTLE SOMETHING" DURING A FAST?

There are many people who balk at the idea of a **complete fast** — that is, going on nothing but water — but might be tempted to try it if only they could eat a small amount of food each day, in order to "keep up their strength." This half-way measure is not to be commended, for two reasons. In the first place, food does not maintain strength in the manner commonly supposed, as we have shown; and, in the second place, such a procedure tends to *keep the patient hungry*. Bear in mind that even *one mouthful* of food tends to break the fast, since it stimulates the stomach into renewed activity and "habit hunger" will be sure to return. It is far easier to go on a complete fast than it is on a partial fast; and after the first two or three days the patient will have no desire for food, which may even seem repulsive to him. This is no cause for alarm, since nature will invariably indicate when food is again wanted, by restoring the natural appetite. Eating "just a little" each day is, in fact, a much greater hardship than abstaining from food altogether. Fasting is not a great strain upon the patient, once he has undertaken it; in fact many people have been surprised to find how easy it is. A reduced diet, or a fruit-juice diet, is all very well, and will doubtless produce beneficial results in the long run; but such measures must not be confused with fasting, and the patient undertaking a real fast would be far better off if he avoided all such measures, and made up his mind to undergo a strict fast instead.

"I love to eat!" How often have we heard this remark — and how low an estimate we form of human nature in consequence! On more than one occasion, when discussing fasting with some friend who was ill, I have heard him make the remark, "I'd rather eat and die than fast and live!" Well, of course, the choice was his, since this is a free country. So the best one can do with such individuals is to leave them alone — and let them die! As a famous physician once remarked to a patient of his: "Well, you've always lived like a hog, and now you're going to die like one!" This book is not written for those who "love to eat;" it is for those who love life!

Much has been written, of late years, on self-realization, self-conquest, renunciation, the attainment of ideals, and so on. I have known many people who live almost ascetic lives, ruled by stern discipline; yet these same individuals eat like pigs! All logical self-discipline starts from within; all mental, physical and moral control begins with this inner control. And it is, I believe, a fundamental truth that the man who can control his stomach can control himself, and that all other discipline emerges from this central control, and will be proportionately easy, once this has been mastered. The man who has "shrunk his stomach" by moderate eating has learned to control his appetite; and the man who has mastered his appetite has made the first and most important step toward mastering himself. This the philosophy of fasting teaches us.

"IF I SKIP A MEAL I GET A HEADACHE!"

How often have I heard people say that if they don't eat at the regular time, or they are forced to skip a meal, they feel weak and giddy, and have a terrific headache! The very fact that the postponement or omission of a meal causes a headache is a sure sign that not one, but a dozen meals should be skipped. A headache of this kind is caused because poisons and waste-matter are suddenly being thrown into the blood stream and, finding their way to the brain, cause the headache in consequence. It is a sure indication that anyone suffering in this way is in need of a fast, in order to get rid of his toxemia. Anyone in relatively normal health does not develop a headache of this kind; he merely gets hungry. If he does not eat, this "habit hunger" passes off, and will not return until he begins to think of food again. When he does, his mouth begins to water, the gastric juices are poured out, and hunger again returns — more insistently than before. . . . But this is not the case if the patient is really *ill*. Then, even the thought of food is repellent to him; any attempt to eat nauseates him. Giddiness and headache, if they develop, are sure indications that a fast of several days is needed — to rid the system of its accumulatd poisons. Eating, at such times, may indeed cause the headache to disappear; but the *causes* of the headache are then allowed to run-on in the body, and the individual may develop some serious sickness in the near future. Fasting should not be blamed for the headache, but rather those casual factors which fasting has brought to the surface and made manifest. It is a warning; a danger-signal, indicating that a period of fasting is desirable. If the fast is persisted in, the headache will soon pass-off, as the various eliminating organs "get busy" disposing of the toxic material which caused it in the first place.

A simple analogy. Take an ordinary sponge. If the sponge is full of water, it fails to soak-up any more water, when placed in it, **because its saturation-point** has been reached. But *squeeze out* the sponge, so that it is nearly dry, and place it in water, and it will immediately soak-up a quantity of the liquid, as we know; and this process may be repeated any number of times.

It is much the same with the human body. If it is surfeited with an excess of food-material, it cannot possibly absorb any more. Further, it cannot eliminate rapidly enough the excess already there. The squeezing-out process corresponds to the fast. By under-nourishing the body for a certain length of time, the various eliminating organs are given a chance to "catch-up," so to say, and get rid of this excess, so that the 'human sponge' is once more in a condition to absorb more water (food), to fill its vacant spaces. . . . The analogy is of course a rough one, but is perhaps simple enough to give one a sort of bird's eye picture of what actually goes on in the body when food is withheld. Fasting merely enables the depurating **organs to eliminate the unused and unwanted excess,** which our previous habits of over-eating have pro-

53

duced. It is, in fact — as I have so often stressed — a simple and efficient form of "house cleaning."

"COLDS"

The old and popular delusion — that you must "stuff a cold and starve a fever" — has done inestimable harm. . . . The real meaning of the old adage is: "*if* you stuff a cold, you *thereby* have to starve a fever." As a matter of fact, all colds are accompanied by fever. A cold is a clear indication that the body is choked and blocked with an excess of waste material and toxins, which the system endeavors to dispose of in every way possible — being poured out on the mucous surfaces in great quantity. The proper procedure is to place the patient upon a fast immediately, keeping him warm — and preferably in bed. Two or three days' fasting will "cure" the most obstinate cold, as Mark Twain emphasized in one of his serious Essays. [1] Of course the cold itself is really a curative process, and as such cannot be "cured!" However, when food is withheld, the eliminating organs have a chance to rid the system of this toxic load, with the result that the "cold" is soon disposed of. Anyone suffering from a 'cold' can easily prove the truth of these statements by trying it upon himself, and he will find that his trouble will vanish like mist before the morning sun. (See Dr. Haig's *Etiology of a Common Cold*, etc.)

FASTING AND THE PSYCHONEUROSES

It is the all but universal practice to "stuff" all patients suffering from one or other of the psycho-

_____

(1) "*The Appetite Cure*," in his book The Man That Corrupted *Hadleyburg*, etc. See also his "*My Debut as a Literary Person*," in the same volume, which is also a strong defense of fasting.

neuroses; this is thought to constitute an essential element in their treatment, and any gain in weight is held to be a sure indication of their progressive recovery. One reason for this, doubtless, is that excessive eating tends to *smother symptoms* — the genererated poisons acting upon the brain and nervous system like a sedative. If the suppression of symptoms really benefitted the patient, there might be some excuse for this; but we all know that such is not the case; and, while undernourishment may make the patient excited for a time, this would only be temporary, and the ultimate benefits would be manifest in the improvement of the patient's condition. Toxins *must* affect the brain cells adversely, and their elimination *must* benefit them in the long run. We have seen that one of the surest ways of disposing of these toxins is by fasting.

A famous psychiatrist once remarked that "every nervous patient has gas, and when he has a fit of anger he suffers from a gas attack." This is doubtless true. Destructive emotions — such as fear, anger, hatred, etc. — will stimulate the formation of large quantities of gas; but the reverse of this is also true, *viz.*, that *gas will increase the neurosis!* This is a fact which has never been pointed out, so far as I know; but numerous observations prove it to be a fact. The way to reduce the emotions — *and* the neurosis — is to prevent the formation of gas; and this can of course most effectually be done by cleansing the bowels, and placing the patient upon a partial or complete fast. If psychiatrists once realized the true rationale of fasting, they would doubtless be inclined to give it a fair trial in treating the psychoneuroses. The beneficial effects upon the mind which may be noted in all normal persons should furnish a clue to its efficacy in such cases.

FASTING IN CHILDHOOD AND IN SPECIAL CONDITIONS

Fasting may be employed as a therapeutic measure, and with equal benefit, in both acute and chronic diseases. It is usually easier to induce the patient to undertake a fast in the former, for the reason that hunger is absent and even the thought of food may be nauseating. The more severe and serious the condition, the more imperative the fast becomes. The delay of even a few days may be fatal. Place all such patients on a fast at once — and, if need be, argue with them afterwards!

In chronic cases it may be more difficult to induce the patient to fast, unless he understands its philosophy, and knows what he is doing. Fear of the fast must first be disposed of. Once this has been overcome, it may be undertaken with safety, and with greatly added benefit. The patient must really *want* to fast in order to derive the greatest advantages from it.

In cases of extreme emaciation, fasting should be undertaken with caution, and a long fast should not be attempted. Fasts of one or two days may be alternated by days of rational feeding. As the patient gains health and strength, longer fasts may be indulged in. Thin patients often derive great benefit from fasting, and it is a mistake to assume that only the fat and the fleshy can fast with safety. It is only when the emaciation is extreme that the above caution holds good.

Children, even infants, may often fast to great advantage, and so may the aged. The rejuvenating effects of a fast are very apparent in the latter cases. They often add greatly to their vital powers, and years to their lives, in consequence of properly conducted periods of fasting. In lactation, short fasts are also beneficial, and during pregnancy it must not be considered a dangerous expedient. If the prospective mother is really ill, she should not be afraid of fasting any more than at any other time. Long fasts are not of course suggested; but short fasts, alternating with days of light eating, will only benefit the patient, and will facilitate the ultimate delivery.*

The weak and the devitalized should not hesitate to fast, as a rule. Their weakness is due to toxemia — not to the lack of food. In this connection, Mr. Upton Sinclair says:

"There is no greater delusion than that a person needs strength to fast. The weaker you are from the disease, the more certain it is that you need a fast, and the more certain it is that your body has not strength enough to digest the food you are taking into it. If you fast under these circumstances, you will grow not weaker, but stronger. In fact, my experience seems to indicate that the people who have the least trouble on the fast are the people who are the most in need of it. The system which has been exhausted by the efforts to digest the foods that have been piled into it, simply lies down with a sigh of relief and goes to sleep."

Fasting is contra-indicated only in a very small number of cases. In ninety-nine cases out of a hun-

*The old adage that the expectant mother must "eat for two" is of course nonsense. Suppose the baby weighs nine pounds at birth. This is a pound a month, or approximately half an ounce a day! Yet women are urged to eat one or two pounds of additional food, to compensate for this gain! Is it any wonder that they have trouble in child-birth?

dred, only benefit will be noted as the result of a longer or shorter period of fasting.

PREVENTION VS. "CURE"

The old saying that "an ounce of prevention . . ," etc., is never more fully borne-out than in cases of fasting. If the patient had lived abstemiously — maintaining a physiological balance between income and outgo, insofar as his food was concerned — no period of fasting would have been necessary; a normal state of health would have been preserved, and the condition requiring such radical treatment prevented. It must not be forgotten that fasting is only advocated in distinctly abnormal conditions — when symptons develop indicative of a so-called "disease." Thus applied, it has great potency. But it would be far more sensible to prevent the onset of this condition in the first place, by right living, and thus obviate the unpleasant consequences which ensue —- including the fast! A frugal diet, coupled with other hygienic conditions, would have insured this.

PART IV

FOOD AND DIET

THE QUESTION OF DIET

Food may be considered from two standpoints: that of *quantity* and that of *quality*. With the former of these questions the present book is mainly concerned. It is my belief that the vast majority of people over-eat, thereby making themselves ill, necessitating the fasting treatment herein advocated. But it must never be forgotten that, if people limited themselves to the right amount of food, these conditions would never arise — and hence no fasts would be necessitated. It is only in cases of illness that fasting is advocated; it then becomes a therapeutic measure. At all other times we must of course eat regularly — though sparingly! It is the *excess* of food which causes the harm. I have already covered this aspect of the subject in various sections of this book.

Food should of course be thoroughly masticated — especially carbohydrates. The reason for this is that chewing the food is not merely a mechanical process, for the purpose of breaking-down the food into small particles; it is also a chemical process, since the saliva is alkaline, and the initial stages of digestion (for all carbohydrate foods) must take place in an alkaline medium. The digestive juices of the stomach are acid; so that, if these substances are not converted in the mouth, they have to wait until they reach the intestines (also alkaline), with the result that they ferment, creating gases which are very troublesome. Thorough mastication of such foods is therefore essential. Further, such a procedure enables us to be satisfied with less food — always an advantage.

More and more the general public is accepting the idea that fruits, salads, simple vegetables, etc., constitute the most wholesome diet, and that excessive sweets, fats and starches in any form are detrimental.

Vegetarians have long contended that meat is not only unnecessary, but harmful. Meat is undoubtedly a highly stimulating and toxic food. Until relatively recently, it was also a "luxury." Only the rich could afford meat with any regularity. The question often raised — as to whether man 'can live' without meat is of course ridiculous, in view of the fact that the majority of the human race have always done so, and that a large percentage of them still do! Many of the world's greatest thinkers have been vegetarians — and have enjoyed exceptionally long lives and good health. Meat is certainly not a necessary food; and there is much evidence showing that the human race would be far better off without it.

Fruit on the other hand is not merely an adjunct to food, but should be eaten *instead* of other food; not in addition to it, but in place of it. There are thousands of persons who live on a 'fruitarian' diet — that is, fruits and nuts alone, uncooked and in a natural state; and many books have been written in defense of this diet (See e.g., the present writer's book, *The Natural Food of Man*). Minerals. vitamins, and other essentials are supplied by these foods, which are lacking in the ordinary "mixed" diet. But without at the present time stressing this view, it is certainly true that fruits should constitute an essential part of all normal and healthful regimens.

The quality of our food is therefore extremely important, and every sensible person should inform himself upon this question, by personal experimentation and by reading several good books upon the subject. Many such books are now on the market, dealing with the relative values of foods — as well as with their combination — and the question of hygienic cookery. I would refer the reader to such works —

since I have no space to deal with these questions in the present volume.

ELIMINATION DIETS

Many contend that it is not really necessary to go on a strict fast, since the same results can be obtained by special diets — such as milk, grapes, grape-juice, fruit juices, etc. In certain cases, such diets may be indicated, and will prove highly beneficial, and it is true that great benefit may often be derived from such diets, especially if they are followed for some considerable period of time. It should be pointed out, however, that the bowels are never really emptied, as they are during a fast, and that the digestive organs are not given the rest they would have, were food withheld altogether. But, in chronic cases, such diets are often valuable.

It is in severe acute cases that the fast is most imperative, and then there should be no half-way measures, since the life of the patient is really endangered. The sicker the patient, the more imperative does an immediate and complete fast become. It is in these cases that the powerful effects of fasting are most clearly noticeable. For those who have the necessary confidence in this method, and the will power to carry it through, no diet can equal the complete fast in its efficacy. It is only when this is contra-indicated, for some reason or other, that an elimination diet should be substituted instead. Of these, fruit juice is undoubtedly the best.

HOW ABOUT MINERAL AND
VITAMIN DEFICIENCY?

One objection has been raised to fasting which seems at first sight to possess some degree of validity.

This is that, when the body is deprived of food, it draws upon its own stored reserves, and may quite possibly develop a deficiency "disease" in consequence, since the vitamins and valuable mineral-salts in the body would thereby be drawn upon, with no means for their replenishment.

This topic is one which has been dealt with at considerable length by several of the newer writers on therapeutic fasting, and shown by them to be an objection devoid of validity. Doctor Shelton, e.g., in his *Hygienic System* (Vol. 3) says in part:

"We have no means of knowing how much of a reserve store of vitamins the body possesses, nor do we know where all these reserves are stored . . . But we may be sure of one thing, namely, that these stores are sufficient to outlast the most prolonged fast. We know that rickets is positively benefitted by fasting. We know that scurvy and beri-beri never develop on a fast . . . The fasting patient, after a most prolonged fast, not only does not present these or any other nervous symptoms, but has lost all or nearly all of the nervous symptoms he may have had at the beginning of the fast. Almost all the effects of fasting . . . are exactly opposite to the effects of the deficient or denatured diet . . . if it could be shown that fasting ever produces 'deficiency disease,' then this objection would have some weight. As it is, all the facts of experience must silence the voice of this theory."

Doctor Weger again says:—

"Even though vitamins are consumed in a small degree by fasting, we consider this factor quite negligible compared with the refinement of body chemistry and the overwhelming influences for general good that take place. After a fast the tissues are receptive and readily assimilate as well as utilize vitamins that are necessary elements contained in vital or base-forming foods.''

Cases of real malnutrition or 'deficiency diseases' have never been noted in cases of therapeutic *fasting* — though they may well have been observed in cases of *starvation*. Objections to this method of treatment are invariably based upon the confusion of these two terms; but, as we have seen, there is all the difference in the world between them, and no hygienist ever advocated starvation! Fasting, properly conducted, does not produce this condition, and the patient undergoing a fast need therefore have no fear of it.

PART V

HELPS WHILE FASTING

EXERCISE — DURING THE FAST

It is everywhere acknowledged that the more physical labor a man does, the more food he requires; that the more exercise we indulge in the more food we should eat. This is all very well and good. But it is unfortunately true that the vast majority of people, after reaching maturity, take hardly any exercise at all, and yet eat like horses! Why all this food, if only a very small quantity of the bodily tissue is broken down by physical exertion?

The answer is, of course, that there is no need for it at all. We eat merely to satisfy our appetites, and because we like eating! It is not necessary. People living a sedentary life should eat very little food; yet they eat as much as a man doing a hard day's labor. This excess must cause trouble. The body becomes clogged and poisoned with the excess, and sickness results, How much exercise is taken during sickness? Practically none at all, as we all know. Often, the patient lies in bed for days at a time, without even getting out of bed. How much bodily tissue can be broken down at such times Virtually none! And yet many doctors insist that the patient should be "well fed" at such times, in order to "keep up his strength." How ridiculous, in view of the equivalence which is everywhere acknowledged as being necessary, when the patient is in normal health! If no body-tissue is broken down, surely none is in need of replacement. Yet the poor patient is often stuffed with food regardless.

Inasmuch as the fasting cure is largely a rest cure, too much exercise must be avoided, as a rule, while the fast is in progress. Strenuous activity is certainly *tabu*. The patient should rest in bed whenever he feels so disposed, and plenty of sleep and relaxation are essential. The more he can free himself from worries and tensions the better.

I have known patients who indulged in a certain amount of active exercise every day throughout a long fast, feeling stronger and more vigorous as the days passed. I myself have seen patients who were so "weak" at the beginning of the fast that they could hardly walk up stairs, yet — after twenty or thirty days of nothing but water — were walking five and six miles a day with ease! In their cases, obviously, their weakness was the result of their toxemia and, as these poisons were removed from their systems, greater energy was manifested in consequence. Their weakness was due to their disease, not to the absence of food; and as their systems were cleansed and purifid, by the fast, their vital energies returned — being utilized, however, in the ever-increasing rapidity of the elimination-process. [1]

If the patient is well and strong, a certain amount of active exercise may well be permitted; but it must be remembered that the majority of persons undergoing a fast are weak, ill and devitalized, and in no condition to expend their energies recklessly, in strenuous physical exertion. Their energies are already at a low ebb, and must be hoarded carefully, so that they may be directed to the business of "house cleaning." After all, the fast is really a *rest cure* — a rest for the internal organs normally expending an enormous amount of energy in the conversion and digestion of great masses of food. In general, it may be said that if the patient feels well and strong, and craves exer-

(1) An interesting analogy might be drawn here. Dr. Hampson, in his book *Radium Explained*, remarked that—"the only way yet discovered of influencing the output of energy by radium is simply to increase the activity of the material by purifying it . . . " (p. 64).

cise, he may take a certain amount of it; if he does not, he should rest and not force himself to undertake any strenuous physical activity.

AIR AND BREATHING

Deep breathing exercises two or three times a day are beneficial to anybody, and the same is true during a fast. Plenty of fresh air should be allowed in the room, both day and night. If the air at night is cold, the patient should be wrapped-up warmly and have plenty of bed covers, to prevent him from becoming chilled. Night air is as healthful as it is in the day time, and the old superstition that night air is to be avoided because it is cold and damp has long since been discarded. Cool, fresh air is essential at night.

Breathing should be through the nose, since this filters, moistens and warms the air before it reaches the lungs. If you have a tendency to breathe through the mouth, there is something wrong with you. Possibly the nasal passages are blocked by catarrh. Such a condition is quickly cured by fasting, however, and its beneficial effects will be noted almost immediately. Tension of any kind will have a tendency to cause you to hold your breath; relaxation will facilitate deep, easy breathing. Clearance of any lung trouble is one of the first things noted during a fast.

CLOTHING

The fasting patient must be kept warm! For this reason bed is a good place for him, especially during the winter time, and if the house is not well heated. There should be plenty of covers on the bed — as the surface of the body must not be allowed to become chilled.

When the patient dresses, warm underclothing and

thick suits (or dresses) should be worn; and in winter time the hands and feet should be well protected. The clothing should be loose, to allow a plentiful supply of air to the surface of the body. It should not be too heavy. Aside from this, any ordinary clothing may be worn. In summer time, of course, the clothing may be adjusted accordingly; but if the evenings are cool, a change to heavier clothing should be made. The patient should feel free to go to bed whenever he feels like doing so.

BATHING

During a fast, the skin becomes increasingly active, and its efforts at elimination should be assisted by fairly frequent bathing. Warm and hot baths are helpful, followed by a cool shower, to close the pores of the skin and prevent the sensation of cold. Cold baths or showers in the winter are not advised, unless the patient is robust, and has been used to them for years. The skin must be kept clean and active, since this helps materially in the process of elimination. Beyond this, the bathing habits should be normal, and in conformity with the usual daily life.

WATER DRINKING

How much water should one drink while fasting? This is a question which has been much discussed by those who have had experience in this field. Some contend that very little should be drunk, and others that large quantities should be imbibed, in order to flush the system and assist in elimination. Certainly water should be drunk whenever thirst is present, and it is also true that the drinking of water will serve to offset the gnawing sensations in the stomach which may be experienced during the first few days of the fast.

Whenever these are felt, a glass of water should be drunk, and the attention immediately diverted to something else . . . The value of a *hobby* is nowhere more evident than in these early days, when there is a certain feeling of "loss," by reason of the lack of 'breaks' in the day which meals formerly provided. The busier and more fully occupied you are, during these first few days, the better.

It is probably safer to drink a little too much rather than too little water, during a fast. Pure water never hurt anyone; it enters the system as water and leaves it as water — carrying with it certain salts and waste material . . . However, there is no need to water-log the body, as many believe. A quart a day would probably be a minimum, and three quarts a maximum. Anything between these is allowable, according to the degree of thirst present. More will be craved in summer than in winter.

The sense of taste will probably become so acute, during a fast, that water which normally appeared tasteless now seems to possess a decidedly unpleasant flavor. The purest of water should therefore be provided; and if this still tastes unpleasant, two or three drops of lemon juice may be added to the water, to remove its "flat" taste. More than this is not permissible.

THE PSYCHOLOGY OF FASTING

No one pretends that fasting is a pleasant experience. But if the patient can be made to see that he is *really getting well,* he will persist in it with enthusiasm. He will balance his present minor discomforts against the long period of aches and pains, and perhaps serious illnesses, which preceded it; and if he can be convinced that this procedure will really and truly prevent their recurrence in the future, this will provide him with an incentive to continue the fast, despite its temporary inconveniences. And it must never be forgotten that many people feel much better, both mentally and physically, during a fast than they have for a long time preceding it. Aside from what the fast will do for them, in the future, they see what it is doing for them now — in the immediate relief of many of the pains and difficulties they were formerly experiencing.

It must be admitted that fasting is, in one sense, a *bore* — for those not bedridden and seriously ill. That is perhaps one of his greatest hardships. When it comes to dinner time, and there is no dinner, one feels at first *lost,* with nothing to do — with no break in the day, which the meal formerly provided. Everyone suffers from this, to a greater or lesser extent. It is only natural that they should. The thing to do, at such times, is to drink a glass of water, and *immediately* get busy on something, so as to distract the mind and keep it occupied, until the meal-time has passed. If this can be done it will bridge-over the aching void.

It is also true that thoughts of food will frequently occupy the mind — especially during the first and last days of fasting. Special dishes, or articles of diet, will come to mind; and one cannot help looking forward to the day when they may once again be eaten! But, curiously enough, once the fast is fairly launched, all such ideas vanish, and food offers no temptation. Many fasting patients have sat at the table with their families, and felt no temptation whatever to eat. The thoughts of food during the early days of the fast are due to the mental factor involved in "habit-hunger;" those during the last days are indicative of the growing desire of the body for food, which the return of natural hunger will soon satisfy. They are like the dreams we often experience just before waking. But during the fast itself these thoughts and cravings are rarely experienced; in fact, an actual aversion for food is frequently noted. Needless to say, this aversion disappears with the return of natural hunger, when the fast is ready to be broken.

One's relatives and friends are often most trying, when a fast is undertaken. They keep insisting what a fool the faster is, what dreadful things will surely happen to him, they keep urging him to eat, telling him how thin and ill he looks, and that he will surely ruin his health or lose his mind if he persists in his "crazy" ideas. In short, they make life as miserable as possible for him, by giving him the worst possible sort of suggestions, and urging him to eat, "to keep up his strength." One can only overcome these negative suggestions and this ignorant stupidity by dogged determination — and by thoroughly understanding the philosophy of the fasting cure. If this is fully grasped, no amount of persuasion or counter-argument will be strong enough to shake one's conviction or swerve one from the temporary path he has made up his mind to follow.

No one undergoing a fast should be ashamed of lying down for a certain length of time each day, or of staying in bed for as long as he feels like doing so. Remember, first, that the fasting cure is largely a *rest* cure, and that all rest-cures call for a certain amount of quiescence. Secondly, that the body is undergoing a radical and drastic cleansing process, which is new to it, and that all convalescents are entitled to long periods of rest and relaxation. If you were recovering from a broken leg, or typhoid fever, no one would think it at all "queer" that you spent your time in bed, while recovering; and the same applies to fasting patients, who are in a sense "convalescents." They are recovering from some former illness — which rendered the fast necessary. It is only natural, therefore, that a certain amount of time should be spent in bed. But it must be understood that this is not necessitated by the "weakness" induced by the fast, but by reason of the toxic condition of the body, which has completely devitalized it. Many forms of treatment are accompanied by rest; and fasting is no exception to this rule. It is merely part and parcel of the cure.

The great point is that every patient undergoing a fast should keep his mind occupied, and away from the body. Thinking of food will tend to stimulate the flow of the digestive juices — which is precisely what we wish to avoid. Whenever the thoughts turn in this direction, a glass of water should be drunk, and the mind immediately diverted in other directions.* Premature breaking of the fast may often be prevented by these means. The patient should endeavor to remain happy, cheerful, and confident throughout the fast; he should keep "lifted up" in his mind. If he can succeed in doing this — knowing that the fast is really curing him — he will be enabled to pass through this period with ease and increasing energy and comfort.

THE ENEMA

This is another topic upon which authorities disagree. Dr. Dewey, Dr. Shelton, and others are against the use of enemas, during a fast; while many

*Mahatma Gandhi: "You must cease to think of food whilst you are fasting." (Ethics of Fasting, p. 31).

others are in favor of them. Should enemas be employed — and if so, how frequently?

There can be no doubt that the bowels continue to harbor a surprising amount of "waste," even during a prolonged fast. I have known many patients who took enemas daily, during thirty and forty day fasts, and removed quantities of material every time they took them. It is true that these individuals were in every case large, well-fed persons, who were greatly over-weight. In their cases, certainly, the enemas seemed justified — even necessitated. Thin persons are usually constipated, and the faeces, while less copious, are harder. The "plug" in the rectum should certainly be removed, in all such persons, so that a normal action of the bowels may be possible, without straining. Salt-water enemas are advisable in most cases of constipation and diarrhoea.

Many prepare themselves for a fast by a few days of fruit-diet, just before the fast. This serves the double purpose of loosening the bowels and avoiding the sudden "let-down," which the cessation of food often produces. I have known of others who prepared themselves by taking a dose of Senna leaves, which have a strong laxative action. Nothing of this sort may be taken by way of the mouth during a fast, of course. Anything entering the stomach and stimulating it into activity will have the effect of causing the return of hunger, and thus virtually breaking the fast. All such measures, if taken at all, must be before the fast is entered upon.

The purpose of the enema, of course, is to wash-out the rectum and lower bowel, and assist in the elimination of the waste material which they contain. It is a process of internal hydro-therapy. There is no doubt that the bowels can go for many days without moving, during a fast, and that they will move naturally soon after it is broken; and, as I have said, Dr. Shelton and others are opposed to the enema, while the fast is in progress. He has had great experience with fasting, and his opinion in this matter should, I feel, be given due weight. Nevertheless, I feel that enemas are sometimes of great benefit in fasting cases, inasmuch as they tend to shorten the fast by disposing of the retained waste more quickly. Certainly they can do no *harm*. In many cases they seem to provide relief and prove of great benefit. I am still of the opinion, therefore, that enemas have their place in the fasting treatment — though perhaps not to the degree that many of us formerly supposed.

Enemas, if taken, should not be too copious, and the water should be tepid to cool, so as to stimulate the activity of the bowel. They may be taken, to best advantage, immediately before the fast, and during the first two or three days, and only occasionally thereafter. If the bowels do not move fairly promptly, after the fast is broken, an enema will stimulate them into renewed activity. The water should be retained as long as possible before expulsion, so as to soften the faecal matter and carry-away as much of it as possible, when the water is expelled.

THE MENTAL FACTOR IN FASTING

I have elsewhere emphasized the fact that, while it is virtually impossible — physiologically — to starve to death in less than sixty days, at the least, many people have actually died within a week or two, when lost in the jungle, and completely deprived of food. This is undoubtedly due to the mental factor involved. If a person knows nothing of fasting, and believes that he will die within a few days if he doesn't eat, he may actually do so — or suffer the tortures of the damned. If, on the other hand, he understands the philosophy of fasting, and really *wants* to fast, he will feel well and energetic at the end of the same length of time, and derive only benefit from this priod of abstinence. It's all in the mind! To derive the greatest benefit from a fast, a person must understand it, and "want to fast more than he wants to eat." If he can once attain this mental attitude, half the battle is won.

PART VI

EFFECTS OF FASTING ON THE BODY

THE TONGUE AND THE BREATH

During a fast, the tongue coats heavily and the breath becomes foul. These are sure indications that the elimination of poisons from the body is proceeding at a rapid rate. Every avenue and channel is seized upon, in an effort to dispel the accumulated poisons as rapidly as possible. The mucus coating of the throat and tongue are both utilized, in this expulsive effort.

It must not be forgotten that the condition of the tongue indicates the condition of the mucus membrane throughout the whole alimentary canal. As Dr. Harvey stated, in his work *On Corpulence in Relation to Disease* "The state of the mucus membrane of the tongue indicates the condition of that of the stomach and the intestinal canal." If the tongue is badly coated, therefore, it means that a similar foul condition exists throughout the body. Such a condition evidently calls for some radical cleansing and eliminative measures. These are most speedily and effectually supplied by fasting.

A patient's tongue may be comparatively clean, when he begins the fast, but it will coat immediately the fast begins. This coat usually lasts throughout the fast — only clearing when natural hunger appears and the fast is ready to be broken. Occasionally it does not clear altogether; but in the majority of cases it does, coincidentally with hunger; and this constitutes one of the positive indications that the fast is now ended and the system ready to receive food.

The breath likewise becomes offensive while the fast is in progress, owing to the fact that the lungs are expelling effete material in this way. Physiologists have often stated — erroneously — that this is due to the consumption of the bodily tissues, which evidently need nourishment! Precisely the reverse of this is the case, however. If this were true, the breath would continue to become more and more foul as the fast progressed; while, as a matter of fact, the breath becomes sweet when the fast is ready to be broken, and coincidentally with the return of natural hunger. The breath is a sort of "organic barometer," which indicates the condition of the patient. So long as it is foul and offensive, the fast must continue; as soon as it becomes sweet, the fast is ready to be broken. Nature thus clearly indicates the natural termination of the fast, and constitutes a valuable counter-check on the strictness and the duration of this period of abstinence.

THE BODILY TEMPERATURE

In so-called "cold blooded animals," the temperature of the body is approximately the same as its environment. In "warm-blooded animals," such as man, the bodily temperature is always the same: 98.4°F. It is an astonishing fact that this remains the same, no matter how hot or how cold the weather may be, owing to the internal control — a sort of organic thermostat which regulates the bodily temperature. When the temperature falls a few degrees, we have sub-normal temperatures; when it rises, fever is indicated. The body can withstand such departures from the normal for only a certain length of time — though sub-normal temperatures may continue for long periods if not excessive. Either of them, however, denotes a departure from the normal.

Physiology teaches us that the temperature of the body is maintained by the oxidation (burning) of food material, which maintains its heat, much as an engine is heated when coal is burned. In my *Vitality*,

Fasting and Nutrition, I advanced reasons for thinking that this simple relationship is not justified, and that — just as an electric current heats a wire when passing through (or along) it, — so the vital energies tend to heat the nervous system and the body generally. However, I shall not stress the point here, assuming for the sake of argument that the currently-held relationship is justified.

When a fast is entered upon, the bodily temperature — whether subnormal or the reverse — slowly but surely returns to normal. If fever is present, this is reduced as the fast progresses. Such a result one might have foreseen. But it may be surprising to many to learn that the temperature also rises, during a fast, until it likewise becomes normal! This has been proved by many observations. Dr. A. Rabagliati, e.g., in his *Air, Food and Exercises,* p. 261, says:

". . . I have raised the temperature of a man who was, besides, thin, emaciated, and attenuated by constant vomiting, lasting for seven years, from 96°F. to 98.4°F., by advising him to fast for thirty-five days. On the 28th day his temperature had risen to normal and remained so."

Doctors Tanner, Shelton, Hazzard, Eales and many others testify to like effect, confirming my own observations. The fast invariably raises or lowers the temperature of the body, until it becomes normal. The feeling of chilliness has nothing to do with the actual temperature; and it has frequently been noted that this will drop when food is eaten — after the fast is broken. If food-combustion were the source of the bodily heat, in the sense commonly supposed, it would be difficult to account for such cases.

Subnormal temperatures are due to the choking and blocking of the body by an excess of food-material, preventing the free circulation of blood within it, and the liberation of its energies. Remove this blocking material, allow a freer distribution of vital energies through the body, and the temperature invariably rises . . . Abnormally high temperatures are of course rapidly reduced . . . We have, therefore, in such cases, another indication of the therapeutic value of the fast; also the proper time for its termination. . . . For the temperature returns to normal — coincidentally with the return of natural hunger.

THE PULSE

The pulse throughout the body corresponds, of course, with the action of the heart, and from time immemorial has been utilized as a method of diagnosis. The average adult pulse, under normal conditions, is slightly more than one pulsation a second. Great variations in this may be noted, however, depending upon the amount of exercise taken, the mental and emotional stimuli, etc. Diet also has an effect upon the frequency of the pulse.

The pulse and the temperature of the body often rise and fall together — though this is by no means invariably the case. Abnormally rapid pulses are sometimes noted in fasting cases, while the temperature remains quite normal. On the other hand, the pulse may be slow and feeble. Such extreme variations are, however, the exceptions rather than the rule. In the majority of fasting cases, the pulse remains at a fairly normal rate; and if the fast be persisted in until the return of natural hunger, there will usually be no serious abnormalities to record. Many so-called "weak hearts" have been permanently benefitted by a fast, — the improvement in its depth and rhythm being particularly noticeable.

LOSS OF WEIGHT

The average loss of weight, during a fast, is about one pound a day. If the fast lasts (say) fifteen days, fifteen pounds will be lost, and so on. The loss is slightly more than this at first, and slightly less towards its close; but this is the *average loss.* Observation of many fasting cases have established this rule.

This means that the body loses this much each day, and consequently that approximately a pound of food a day is necessary, in order to maintain the weight of the body in equilibrium. But instead of this, what do we find? That the average person eats two or three, or even four or five pounds of food a day, under the mistaken impression that it is necessary. This means that the digestive organs have to do an enormous amount of unnecessary work, in order to convert and dispose of this great excess; and all this requires the expenditure of an enormous amount of vital energy. If this energy were free to devote itself to other work, a tremendous amount of extra vitality would be conserved; and this is precisely what *is* noted during a fast.

Most people keep themselves tired and worn-out because of this constant drain upon their vital energies — in digesting and disposing of an excess of food. The very process of digestion requires the expenditure of much vitality; and if it is not used in this way it is free to energize the body. Furthermore, this constant excess of food tends to choke and block the body with an excess of poisons and waste material — which induces the feeling of weakness and lassitude. The usual advice to such people is that they should eat more in order to provide greater "strength." Of course, the effect of this practice is still further to poison and weaken the body. And so on, in a vicious circle, until the body breaks down completely, under the strain, and the subject has a serious illness.

Bear in mind, always, that we gain benefit from our food, *not* in proportion to the amount we eat, but in proportion to the amount we can properly utilize and assimilate! We have all known relatively fat people who eat very little; and thin, emaciated people who eat like horses. These people keep themselves thin by their over-eating. None of the food they eat is properly utilized; it merely chokes and blocks the body, preventing it from deriving benefit from any of the food they eat. They are in a constant state of toxemia. Acidosis is present, and this acid tends to eat-up the fatty tissue, so that it is consumed, instead of feeding the body. The way to make these people gain weight is to see to it that they eat less, and not more, food. By reducing the amount, the digestive organs have a chance to convert it properly, and the body to assimilate it, and when this is done the subject gains weight, normally and healthfully.

Inasmuch as the average loss of weight, during a fast, is only about a pound a day, the average person need have no fear of undertaking a fast on that account. Most people are over-weight, and could well afford to lose a few pounds to advantage. It is the safest and the simplest of all methods of "reducing." After the fast is broken, this weight will be restored — to the extent that such restoration is desirable. The patient need never go back to his former over-weight if he does not want to. If due care be taken of the diet, this excess can always be avoided.

Let us take an example, by way of illustration. A woman weighs 195 pounds — much more than she should. She goes on a fast, and reduces her weight to 145 pounds. (In cases of very fat people, consider-

ably more than a pound a day is lost). After breaking the fast, due care is exercised in the diet, and the
patient does not over-eat. In such case, the weight
gradually increases to (say) 163 pounds, where it
remains. For a large-framed, heavy-boned woman,
this weight might be normal. She has effectually and
scientifically "reduced," down to her normal weight,
and this dangerous and cumbersome excess is not again
accumulated, — if due care be taken of the diet. Many
years have doubtless been added to her life in consequence — to say nothing of the freedom from 'disease'
and the added feeling of well-being which she experiences in consequence.

Thin People. The question has often been raised:
is it safe for thin people to undertake a fast? Are they
not undernourished at present, and would not a fast
be dangerous to such people? The answer is that, in
ninety-nine cases out of a hundred, it is perfectly safe
for a thin person to fast, and they would derive great
benefit from so doing. Usually, to be sure, a long
fast is not necessary in such cases, but benefit will
almost invariably be derived from a shorter fast — and
such individuals will gain weight afterwards, bringing
their weight more nearly to normal than it had been
in years.

The reason for all this is very simple, and easily
understood, when the philosophy of the fasting cure
is once comprehended. The thin man is undernourished, it is true; but this is not due to the fact that he
has not eaten enough (for as we know he often eats
far too much) but is due to the fact that his tissues
are both starved and poisoned by the excess. This is
because the blood, carrying nutrient material, cannot
reach the tissues of the body, for the simple reason
that the tiny blood vessels, which supply them, are

choked and blocked with an excess of material, preventing the free flow of blood through them, and consequently preventing food-material from reaching these affected parts. The way to supply more food to these starving tissues is to open-up the blood-vessels, allowing more blood to flow through them, and consequently more nourishment to reach the obstipated tissues. And this can most effectually be brought about by fasting, which removes this clogging material, thereby allowing a freer circulation, which in turn results in greater nourishment. The patient gains weight accordingly.

Bear in mind, always, that emaciation is nearly always due to the wasting of disease — not to lack of food. A person who is really ill can continue to waste-away, no matter how much food he eats; indeed, he often wastes more rapidly than if he ate no food at all. This conclusively proves that emaciation is due to the lack of ability on the part of the organism to assimilate the food eaten, — rather than to a lack of actual food supplied.

When the excessively thin person begins to fast, therefore, what happens is this: Clogging, waste material is absorbed and removed from the tiny blood vessels, allowing a freer circulation of blood through them; acids and poisons are rapidly eliminated; the digestive organs are given a chance to rest, thereby gaining energy and vitality; the whole system is toned-up, so that it is capable of handling and digesting food, when again permitted. The result of all this is that the abnormal wasting of the body ceases, its energies are increased and, when food is again eaten, it is properly digested and carried to the emaciated parts. Added healthy tissue results in consequence.

The condition of the abnormally thin person is

closely allied to that of the patient suffering from anemia, and a few words on this may help us to understand still more clearly exactly what occurs in cases of emaciation.

Anemia. I cannot do better, perhaps, than to quote in this connection the following words by Dr. A. Rabagliati. He says:

"The anemic girl is in a state of indirect, not of direct, anaemia. Her circulation is really blocked. It is a state which may be called 'constipation of the circulation.' The muscular elements of the vessels, and particularly their transverse fibres, are hypertrophied ,and being, besides, over-stimulated, they go into a state of excessive contraction. The effect of this is to narrow the lumen of the vessels, and to prevent the blood from flowing freely along them, and by this means, of course, a proper supply of blood is prevented from reaching the tissues. The consequence is that the girl appears pale and anaemic, and no doubt is so. But the cause is really an excess of food-supply, which in the first instance caused the muscular elements to hypertrophy, and as the over-circulation of too much food still continued, the hypertrophied transverse muscular fibres contracted and narrowed the lumen of the vessels. The process is really a beautifully adapted provision of Nature to limit the blood-supply to parts which have already been over-nourished, and which would tend to become still further hypertrophied if the nutritive process were carried still further. The process is plainly one of starvation, due to over-repletion, caused by contraction of over-fed muscular fibres. And, obviously, the means of treatment proper to such a state is to restrict the diet until, some of the hypertrophy of the muscular fibres of the vessels having been removed, some of the spasm passes off, and blood flows more freely, and the anaemia is reduced. To recommend more food, as is so often done, is to do the precise opposite of what good treatment demands. The meals ought to be reduced in number and quantity, not increased." [1]

If we understand what happens in such cases, we can understand why it is that emaciated persons would likewise receive benefit from fasting, for their condition is very similar. Such individuals may safely undertake a fast with benefit; and after the fast is broken, and the digestive organs rested and ready to receive food, they will find that they will gain in weight rapidly — since the cause of their former excessive thinness has been removed. Thin persons can fast just as safely as fat ones; and with equal benefit.

Fat People. We have been talking about excessively thin people; now let us consider those who are overly fat.

It is true that Nature has provided women with a certain amount of fatty tissue — more than men. The reason for this, in all probability, is that this can be drawn-upon, in times of famine, to provide the unborn child with nutriment, without unduly wasting the body of the mother. In other words, it is a provision against times of famine. But, in our modern civilization, such times of famine are normally lacking, and the tendency of nearly all people is to overeat, as we have seen, rather than to under-eat. The necessity of any excessive amount of fatty-tissue is therefore done away with.

Instead of this small amount of "padding," however, many women — as we know — become excessively fat, and are constantly going to "reducing parlors" in order to get rid of it! This fat is not only

(1) *Aphorisms*, etc., p. 200.

unsightly, but is positively dangerous, from the point-of-view of health. The heart is called upon to perform much added labor, in pumping the blood through this excess of tissue, and the muscles become flabby and lacking in tone. Indeed, Dr. Charles E. Page goes so far as to say:

"A fat person, at whatever period of life, has not a sound tissue in his body; not only is the entire muscular system degenerated with the fatty particles, but the vital organs — heart, lungs, brain, kidneys, liver, etc., — are likewise mottled throughout, like rust spots in a steel watch-spring, liable to fail at any moment . . . Fat is a disease." [1]

Whenever an athlete goes into training, he sees to it that every ounce of fat is got rid of, and we often hear the remark that a man in the pink of condition "hasn't an ounce of fat on him." If this is an ideal state of health, it should be obvious that an excess of fatty tissue represents so much diseased tissue—and must be disposed of before health is fully regained.

Fat can be gained only in one way: through excessive over-eating. If the body is constantly supplied with a super-abundance of food, particularly fats and carbohydrates, it soon begins to accumulate fat; and this can most logically be disposed of by under-nourishing the body for a time, until this is again absorbed. Every fat person needs a fast—but they are usually the very ones who would never consent to take it! All other measures are merely palliative and half-way; they fail to get at the real cause of the trouble. As Dr. Dewey remarked:

"How simple! Only to fast, no matter if it costs a whole day, a whole week or a whole month, and with absolute safety . . . It is a process that you can

(1) *Natural Cure*, pp. 148-49.

93

push safely well on to the skeleton condition, if you cut the food down. You can determine in advance just what loss of weight is to be reached; for it is simply a problem of endurance and mathematics."

Every excessively fat person, then, is in need of a fast; and when such a person becomes ill, the necessity for the fast becomes all the more imperative. Bear in mind that—*fatty tissue is diseased tissue!*

PHYSIOLOGICAL EFFECTS OF FASTING

As before emphasized, the first two or three days of a fast are the trying ones. They are relatively unpleasant for various reasons: The patient misses his regular meals, with the break and stimulation which they afforded; he tends to become bored, — not knowing what to do with himself at regular mealtimes; he may be a little anxious and nervous (especially if he has never fasted before) wondering what is going to happen next; certain symptoms may develop, which are not altogether pleasant, such as a coated tongue, bad breath, a bad taste in the mouth, slight nausea, dizziness when arising, an 'all gone' feeling in the pit of the stomach, etc. As the fast progresses, these all more or less pass away, or he becomes used to them and disregards them, as he learns to understand their significance. If some of them tend to increase for a while, he understands that this is because elimination is going on at a rapid rate, and that the poisonous material thrown into the blood stream is being carried throughout the body for rapid elimination. Continuance of the fast will soon get rid of these unpleasant effects.

Before discussing other signs and symptoms which may develop while fasting, however, let us consider very briefly the effects of this treatment upon the various organs and tissues of the body.

The *stomach* is, of course, affected immediately when a fast is begun. There is a common error that food is soon passed through the stomach, which is invariably empty a few hours after a meal is eaten. In diseased conditions particularly this is not at all the case, for, owing largely to the lowered vitality — and hence lack of vigorous digestive action — food often remains for hours before it is passed-on, into the bowel. Says Dr. Rabagliati:

"Food is occasionally, or even not infrequently, still in the stomach twenty-four, thirty-six, and even forty-eight hours after it has been taken."

I have personally known of cases in which large quantities of food were ejected at the end of a three days' fast — in spite of profuse water drinking! What state must the stomach of this man have been in to render such a result possible? And in what condition was this man's stomach to receive food? Obviously, such a stomach needs rest, and a thorough cleansing, before more food is taken into it. If food is eaten before the last meal has been digested, trouble is bound to follow. Only fasting will thoroughly empty, cleanse and revitalize this over-worked organ.

Many fear that gastric acidity will develop at such times, for if the acid juices of the stomach continue to be secreted, and no food is supplied for them to work-upon, might they not cause injury — perhaps to the lining of the stomach? I can assure the reader that no such result will be noted — or ever has been noted. When food is not eaten, the digestive juices *are not secreted* — or only in very minute quantities — and only begin to flow again when food is eaten. No harm can possibly come to the stomach, therefore, during a fast — no matter how many days it may be deprived of food.

Some have argued that, if the stomach is allowed to "shrink," it may have difficulty in distending itself again, when food is eaten . . . Also that, if the muscles constituting it are allowed to fall into disuse, they may atrophy — as any unused muscles will. Both these arguments are completely unsound. In the first place, the average person's stomach is vastly *over*-distended, as the result of constant over-eating, and should be permitted to shrink to some extent, to reduce it to its normal size. After this has been done, the stomach will function far more efficiently, and so much food will not be craved in the future — thereby reducing the meals to normal.

Secondly, the muscles of the stomach are not, as a rule, normally worked, but vastly over-worked, and the rest they need is furnished only when food is withheld. Its rest is not the rest of disuse, but the rest of recuperation from over-exertion. Like any tired muscle the stomach seeks relaxation Before putting more fuel on the fire we must first of all remove the ashes and debris, and only when this has been done should we add more fuel — which will then burn brightly, by reason of the internal cleanliness and the 'forced draught' which is possible, once the 'clinkers' are thoroughly cleared.

During a fast, the stomach is cleansed and rested; added tone is given its walls; the character of its secretions is improved; the organ is invigorated and refreshed. This is clearly shown by the ravenous appetite which develops after the fast has been broken! Anyone who has experienced this will be willing to testify that his stomach, far from being weakened and devitalized by the fast, now shows every sign of vigorous activity!

The *lungs,* during a fast, respond with remarkable rapidity, and everyone who has tried this method, when his lungs are choked and blocked with an excess of waste material (which they are attempting to eliminate by means of coughing, etc.) will testify to the extremely effective "clearance" of the lungs as soon as food is withheld. The breath becomes tainted — testifying to the rapid elimination which is going-on through these organs. As the fast progresses, the breath sweetens and all the morbid matter which had resided in the lungs is quickly disposed of. As I stated in my former book on the subject:

"The great sense of freedom which is experienced in the lungs, and the ability to talk and sing with greater clearness and facility, and with greater range and depth of tone than had been experienced, perhaps, in months and years, will amply testify that the lungs are far sounder and more normal than they have been —perhaps ever!"

As one might expect, the *liver* and *kidneys,* during a fast, rapidly dispose of the over-load of toxins and impurities they were formerly called upon to handle, and the vital power greatly increases. The *bowels* gradually become emptied of their solid and gaseous contents, and receive a well-earned rest. Irritating material is removed, by natural action — if not by enemas. The whole intestinal tract will be cleansed and invigorated. As soon as the fast is ended, normal bowel actions will be resumed, and will be continued thereafter — especially if reasonable care be exercised in the diet.

The *heart* is likewise greatly benefitted by the fast. Toxins which formerly irritated it have been removed from the body, fatty tissue has been disposed of; the blood has been purified; and less strain has been placed upon the heart, because of decreased stimulation and the lessened amount of work it is called upon to undertake. (See, in this connection, my remarks on "The Pulse").

The *sexual energies* are generally reduced, during a fast — probably because the vital powers are being employed in the work of elimination. It must be remembered also that the fasting patient is generally a *sick* patient, and his energies have for long been at a low ebb . . . However, this is not invariably the case. and many patients have retained their sexual power throughout a fast, or found that it returned strongly at the end of it, when natural hunger and other symptoms indicated that the fast was completed and ready to be broken. In the long run, fasting will be found to restore sexual vigor to the patient — especially to one who has been depleted and ill for a long time. He will find that he has been given a new lease upon life!

The *secretions* are greatly reduced while fasting — the saliva, gastric juice and intestinal juices flowing in far lesser amounts. The quality is, however, greatly improved. The saliva, it is true, is often tainted and offensive, during the early days of the fast, so that a "bad taste" is noted in the mouth; but, as the fast progresses, this gradually passes away, and entirely disappears by the time the fast is ready to be broken. (See the Section on "The Tongue and the Breath").

The *senses* are all rendered more acute; the eyes become bright and the sense of hearing far keener. Certain types of deafness are often cured completely by a fast — especially those due to blockage of the Eustachian tube by catarrh. Touch, smell and taste are also rendered far keener — the latter being noted when the fast is broken. Foods, which taste delicious, are enjoyed as never before, and their various component tastes are capable of being distinguished.

The *blood,* as one might expect, becomes somewhat thinned, but much purer in quality. Dr. Rabagliati noted that the number of red blood corpuscles is often increased during a fast. The *nervous system* is rendered sensitive and the reactions shortened. The *senses,* as we have stated, bcome more acute. Nervousness, which may be present during the early days of the fast, will disappear as it continues. Much of this is doubtless due to the sudden withdrawal of stimulation, which food afforded; but is also largely mental and emotional in character.

It is an interesting fact that the nervous system has the faculty of feeding itself at the expense of the rest of the body, and that, even in cases where the patient has *starved to death,* there has been no appreciable loss of weight of the nervous system. (Yeo: *Physiology;* Wesley Mills, *Animal Physiology;* etc.) Thus, the most priceless and valuable of our possessions preserves itself intact, even in cases of 'starvation' . . . In cases of therapeutic fasting, the tone of the whole nervous system is vastly improved; and this improvement naturally reflects itself in the *mental life* of the patient. Attention, memory, concentration, association, are all rendered more efficient; the brain becomes clear, and thinking, imagination and the inspirational and spiritual forces in man are quickened to a remarkable degree. It is well known that all those undergoing mystical initiations are ordered to fast, as a necessary part of their curriculum. Christ himself is an example of this fact, when he fasted for forty days in the wilderness. All great spiritual teachers have undergone similar periods of fasting. There are certain types of insanity which would doubtless be greatly benefitted by such a procedure.

The statement is frequently made that fasting will produce *acidosis,* and much has been made of this by those who oppose the fasting treatment. As a matter-of-fact this is entirely untrue — as anyone experienced in fasting cases can testify. This condition may result in cases of *starvation* — an entirely different matter, as I have frequently pointed out. Both Dr. Shelton and Mr. MacFadden — who have treated literally thousands of fasting cases — deny that true acidosis appears in properly conducted fasting cases, and Dr. Rabagliati testified to like effect. My own experience has been similar. Dr. Haig stated that "fasting acts like a dose of alkali." Dr. Weger, who also had great experience in the treatment of such cases, stated:

"Fasting is not and cannot be the cause of acidosis, for the symptom-complex of acidosis is quite common in full-fed, plethoric individuals, in whom the makings of acidosis exist as a result of an over-crowded nutrition." He also states that, when symptoms of acidosis appear, "they are of short duration, and easily overcome without interfering with or curtailing the fast." If it is persisted in, such symptoms will disappear. There need therefore be no fear of such a development, as the result of the fast; in fact, fasting will cure this very condition, which may have been latent in the system for a long time prior to its initiation.

There is no evidence that fasting ever injured the *teeth,* as some have contended; on the contrary, ulcerated teeth have been cured, loose teeth have become tight in their sockets, and many extractions have thereby been prevented. As Dr. Jackson remarked, "the teeth, like the skeleton, appear very resistant to inanition."

The *chemical changes* which take place in the fasting body are many, and of great interest. It has been shown that, while its organic constituents are often greatly reduced (fats, proteins, etc.) its inorganic constituents are carefully preserved — showing that Nature hangs-on to these valuable elements, thereby preventing "deficiency." The body exercises remarkable and wise control of its reserves, in this respect, and no actual "deficiency" is ever noted, as the result of a fast. Dr. Shelton has covered this aspect of the subject very thoroughly in his book on "Fasting."

The net result of therapeutic fasting is its remarkably rejuvenating qualities. The patient is made-over and rendered years younger, both in body and spirit, as the result. He has not only added years to his life but life to his years! He seems, in truth, to have drunk of the Fountain of Youth. If you wish to remain beautiful and young, therefore, undertake a fast, and note the results for yourself! As Dr. Shelton expressed it, in his work upon this subject (p. 114):

"The rejuvenating effect upon the skin is visible to all who have eyes to see. Lines, wrinkles, blotches, pimples and discolorations disappear, the skin becomes more youthful; it acquires a better color and better texture. The eyes clear-up and become brighter. One looks younger. This visible rejuvenation in the skin and eyes is matched by manifest evidences of similar but invisible rejuvenescence throughout the body."

CRISES DURING A FAST

Fasting is an unusual experience — especially for anyone who is undertaking it for the first time — with but slight previous knowledge or experience of the

101

subject. He is apt to think about himself and watch himself closely, and any unlooked-for symptom is likely to be magnified a hundred-fold in his mind, creating a minor mental panic. Should this develop, the patient is apt to undertake unwise self-treatment or, worse still, induce him to break the fast hurriedly — thereby possibly inducing a series of unpleasant symptoms. The thing to do, in all such cases, is to keep your head, remain calm and cool, know that everything is going to come out all right eventually, and continue the fast. If this course be followed, no harm will result. (The importance of understanding the philosophy of fasting before undergoing the experience is thus once again brought home to us.)

A *feverish* condition is sometimes noted, during a fast — due doubtless to the fact that elimination is proceeding at a rapid rate and toxic material is being thrown into the blood stream. This need cause no alarm, and will disappear automatically in a short time, as the fast continues. More important is a feeling of *chill*. I have before emphasized the necessity of keeping fasting patients warm; and if they feel cold, or suffer a chill at any time, the best thing to do is to pack them off to bed, with plenty of warm covers, and if necessary a hot water-bottle to the feet. The fasting patient should at all times dress warmly, especially in cold weather, or if it is damp and penetrating. Hot water drinking — instead of cold — may be advisable in some cases.

One symptom often noticed is a feeling of *dizziness* upon arising from a prone position. This will soon pass off, and is no cause for apprehension. The head may be lowered for a few moments, as in cases of threatened fainting; but beyond this no special treatment is called for.

Latent conditions, long dormant, may come to the surface at times, and manifest their presence. This merely shows us that such conditions were never really *cured* — only the symptoms suppressed when originally treated. The continuation of the fast will effectually dispose of these symptoms, just as it would have, if they became manifest for the first time. They indicate that the patient is really getting better, not worse, and that the original trouble is at last being really eradicated.

Cramps, retention of the urine, and *diarrhoea* are conditions occasionally met with during a fast — but most infrequently. If they develop, the fast should be continued, and hydrotherapeutic measures taken — such as hot compresses, sitz baths, enemas, etc. Gentle massage is often very useful in such cases. *Fainting* should be treated as it is at any other time.

Headaches sometimes develop — more often during the first two or three days, but occasionally later on in the fast. They are doubtless due to the toxic material poured into the blood stream, and carried to the head. Rest and sleep, cool cloths to the head, stroking and suggestion, may all be employed to advantage in such cases. They are almost invariably of short duration, and need cause no more worry than they do at any other time. A 'bad taste in the mouth' may be relieved usually by gargling the mouth and throat with a mild solution of salt and water.

Insomnia may occasionally develop during a fast — though many patients sleep more than usual. A prolonged warm bath will usually produce relaxation and sleepiness. The important thing, however, is the avoidance of *worry* on the part of the patient — since it has been shown that worry about loss of sleep is far more injurious than the loss of sleep itself. The fasting patient is probably taking but little exercise, while his internal organs are also resting, since they are not being called upon to handle and digest food, ordinarily supplied. Relatively few toxins are being created within the body. Under the circumstances, it is only natural that fewer hours of sleep should be called for; so that the patient is not really suffering from insomnia at all, but simply requires less sleep. No worry should be felt, therefore, if less than the usual number of hours are spent in slumber. However, should sleep be craved, this should by all means be allowed — since it indicates in this case a state of exhaustion, due to disease and fatigue resulting from previous habits of life. Rest and relaxation can hardly be overdone, during a fast.

Palpitation is a disagreeable symptom, which may occasionally develop. This may be occasioned by physical or by emotional causes, or by both. Fear and anxiety will quickly produce this symptom — just as they do in normal life. If the patient has a mental panic, his heart will palpitate. The more it palpitates the more fearful he will become; and the more fearful he becomes the more his heart will palpitate! He is in a vicious circle, which must be broken. We often notice the same state in patients suffering from some form of psychoneurosis — fear-cases especially — in which one of the commonest fears is that they are going to die of "heart disease!" No amount of reassurance will satisfy such patients, who often go from one heart specialist to another, only to be assured by every one of them in turn that "there is nothing wrong with your heart." This is doubtless true, insofar as the organic condition of the heart is concerned; anatomically the organ is perfectly sound. But functionally it is misbehaving; and it is palpitating as it does because of the patient's inner emotions — fear and worry. Relieve these, and the palpitation ceases at once. It is a purely temporary and functional condition.

The same is true in fasting cases, when the patient begins to be apprehensive over his condition, because of the appearance of some minor and unexpected symptoms, which he may not fully understand. The thing to do, in such cases, is to calm the patient's fears and reduce his emotions; and this may be done by explaining to him, cálmly and clearly, just what is happening, and getting him to see that the palpitation he notices has been induced by his own mental and emotional states, is purely functional in character, and is not dangerous. Suitable "suggestions" may follow this explanation, calculated to soothe and quiet him, and induce a state of relaxation and (if possible) sleep. Freedom from internal tension will immediately relieve this condition, if brought-on by emotional disturbances — as it is in the majority of cases.

Physical conditions may at times play their part, though in a minor degree. If there is gas in the stomach, this should be assisted to escape, since a distended stomach may press upon the heart. Many deaths from "heart failure" are doubtless due to this cause — following "acute indigestion." A prone position and relaxation will usually allay such unpleasant symptoms.

If the *pulse* is abnormally *slow*, a hot bath will often prove of great value. If the patient is feeling well and strong, gentle exercises, deep breathing, etc., may well be undertaken to advantage. An abnormally *rapid pulse,* on the other hand, may again be due to emotional causes, or some physical condition. Relaxation, suggestion, baths, etc., are helpful in such cases also. Tensions of any kind, physical or mental, must be removed. The above measures will go far to insure this.

Vomiting is perhaps the most serious condition that can develop during a fast. If this occurs during the first day or two, no special apprehension need be felt, but if it is after the fast has continued for some time, prompt action should be taken. The drinking of hot water, hot compresses, spinal manipulations, placing the hands over the pit of the stomach, etc., will often cause the cessation of vomiting. A prone position and relaxation are generally beneficial. Above all, the patient must be soothed and prevented from getting into a panic, because of this untoward symptom. If his emotions are reduced and his fears calmed, half the battle will be won.

In the majority of cases of vomiting, the rule holds good: do not allow the patient to break the fast! If he continues fasting, this condition will pass off, and he will often feel much better afterwards in consequence. In rare cases, it may be permissible to break the fast — especially if the patient feels weak and has fasted for some time. If this is found necessary, the utmost care must be exercised in breaking it gradually and wisely, so as to avoid unpleasant reactions and the continuance of the vomiting. This condition has rarely been noted in fasting cases; but it has occasionally been seen, and when it occurs the advice should be sought, if possible, of one thoroughly conversant with fasting cases.

Very few deaths have ever been recorded, during a fast, and these have been in those cases when the patient was already at his "last gasp" before the fast was undertaken. In all the cases treated by Dr. Dewey, he had in all only five deaths, and these were all of the character indicated above. Whenever a cure is possible

106

at all, fasting will effect it. Thousands upon thousands of patients have undergone the fasting treatment, during the past few decades, and in practically all cases with great benefit. The average person need have no fear on that score, therefore.

Death may well occur in starvation, it is true; but if the distinction between fasting and starvation be kept in mind, it will be realized that the dangers attendant upon starvation are not present in therapeutic fasting — which in practically all normal cases will be found to be the greatest and most potent remedial agent known to man. As Dr. Dewey so truly said: "Take away food from a sick man's stomach, and you have begun — not to starve the sick man, but the disease." There is the whole science and philosophy of fasting in a nutshell.

The patient undertaking a fast should realize that the symptoms noted above, while they have been observed in exceptional cases, are *very rare,* and that the vast majority of people pass though a fast without experiencing any of them. They are mentioned merely for the sake of completeness, and to indicate what should be done, in case one or more of them should develop. Most fasts proceed smoothly and easily, with no unpleasant consequences. Nature is healing the patient as rapidly as he can be healed, and occasional crises which may develop are largely indications that such drastic curative action is being undertaken. Many people feel better during a fast than they have felt in years. The beneficial after-effects are often astounding. The patient will feel that he has taken a new lease on life, as the rejuvenating effects of the fast become evident in renewed vigor and greater vitality. He will in very truth be "born again."

HOW TO BREAK THE FAST

When the time comes to break the fast, Nature will invariably let you know — by a series of unmistakable symptoms. The most important of these is the return of natural hunger, which had been lacking before. The smell and taste of food now appeal to you; your mouth begins to water when thinking of it, and your stomach will indicate its desire for food by a genuine craving—a real sense of hunger. Bear in mind that this sensation is, as a rule, entirely lacking throughout the fast: it disappears after the second or third day, and does not again return until the body is ready for food. When it returns, it is a sure sign that your fast has been satisfactorily completed, and that your body now craves nourishment.

Coupled with the return of natural hunger, other symptoms are noted. The breath (which hitherto had been offensive) sweetens; the tongue becomes clean, ridding itself of its whitish "coat." A sense of re-juvenation and well being returns. The simultaneous appearance of these symptoms is an indication that your fast has terminated, and that you may now eat.*

It is impossible for anyone to say, beforehand, just how long a fast should be. Nature will always deter-mine that. In some cases, only four or five days may be necessary; in others twenty days, in still others five or six weeks or longer, and so on. No one should say, therefore, "I am going on a ten day fast," — or what-ever length of time he has decided upon. Premature

---

*A word of warning should be given here. While it is true that, in a good ninety percent of cases, the tongue clears completely, this is not invariably the case; in certain in-stances a slight coat remains, and the patient must not be obstinate enough to continue his fast until this coat dis-appears. If natural hunger returns, he should break his fast regardless; otherwise he is liable to starve himself—a very different thing from therapeutic fasting, as I have repeatedly emphasized.

breaking of the fast, or prolonging it after it should be terminated, are both harmful, and must by all means be avoided. If the patient's system requires a twelve day fast, and it is artificially broken at the end of the tenth day, trouble is bound to result. The patient may become giddy and nauseated, and be forced to vomit the food he has eaten. This violent reaction will often create a mental panic, causing no end of harm. Whenever this occurs, the subject must immediately resume his fast, and determine not to break it until clear indications are given that natural hunger has returned and that the body is now ready for food. Disregard of this point constitutes the chief danger, in all fasting cases.

If you decide to undertake a fast, therefore, do not determine beforehand how long this will be. Be content to go along from day to day, with no definite time-limit in view. Determine to fast as long as necessary, now that you have undertaken it, and get it over with once and for all. Do not break the fast prematurely, just because a certain number of days have elapsed. One thought you may find helpful in this connection is this: Analyze your own immediate bodily sensations, and say to yourself, "Do I feel weak or ill at this particular moment?" Invariably you will find that you are feeling all right *now;* what you are really fearing is that you won't be feeling so spry an hour hence — or the next day! But this is anticipated fear — borrowing trouble in advance. For, when the time comes, you will find that you are feeling all right then too, and that you have had all your worry for nothing. If you can make yourself run along in this manner, from hour to hour and from day to day, you will find that the fasting period becomes much easier, and that your worries and apprehensions will vanish, leaving you confident and encouraged as you proceed.

Premature breaking of the fast is therefore the greatest danger to be avoided. If this is done, and unpleasant consequences ensue, the fast should be resumed until these have subsided, and natural hunger returns. It may then be safely broken without any unpleasant after-effects.

The undue prolongation of the fast is also to be avoided. Once hunger has returned, food must be eaten; if not, starvation begins — which no one would recommend. This brings us to the much misunderstood question of the difference between fasting and starvation — which most people erroneously confuse. This difference may be defined as follows: *Fasting begins with the omission of the first meal and ends with the return of natural hunger; starvation begins with the return of natural hunger and ends in death.* The former is a beneficial, therapeutic measure, resulting only in benefit to the patient; the latter is destructive and harmful. Where the one ends, the other begins. This book deals only with therapeutic fasting.

The question now arises: When the fast is ready to be broken, what should the patient eat? What food should be allowed, and how often and how much? These are very important questions, since the improper breaking of the fast — especially if of fairly long duration — will often result in trouble, and offset much of the good which the fast has brought about. It is therefore a matter of no little moment. Let us see what the best authorities have to say on this subject.

The general opinion of those who have made studies of fasting cases is that the first "meal" should consist of a glass of orange juice and water. This should not be too cold, and should be taken slowly, in

110

sips. If it is drunk too rapidly, it is liable to result in cramps and the formation of gas. Sipped slowly, these unpleasant symptoms are avoided. From three to five minutes should be consumed in drinking this glass of diluted orange juice. Each sip should be "chewed" before being swallowed. In this way the acid of the fruit is mixed with the saliva, and the reaction in the stomach reduced to a minimum.

Some three hours after this, all being well, a second glass of diluted orange juice may be taken — the percentage of fruit juice being slightly higher. If the fast is broken in the afternoon or evening, nothing more should be taken that day. If, however, it is broken in the morning, or the early part of the day, a first "meal" may be taken around the usual dinner-time in the evening.

Regarding the composition of this first meal, opinions differ. Some are in favor of warm milk; others of well-cooked mashed vegetables; others of tomato juice; others of a thick soup—thoroughly masticated; others of a poached egg on whole wheat toast, with a cup of warm milk. I have observed good results in all these cases, and there is probably little to choose between them. (Of course if the patient possessed an "allergy" for eggs before the fast, one of the other meals should be taken). The main thing is that this first meal *must* be small, and it *must* be eaten slowly and masticated thoroughly. Nothing more should be allowed the first day.

It must be remembered that, as soon as the fast is fairly broken and hunger returns, the patient is likely to develop a ravenous appetite during the ensuing days. It is most essential that this be controlled. Overeating during the days immediately following a fast will often result in complications, and undo much of the benefit derived from the treatment. The appetite *must* be controlled for the first few days following a fast! And the longer the fast has been, the greater the care that must be exercised.

After the first day, the foods usually eaten may be resumed, but in small quantities and eaten slowly. Not more than two small meals should be allowed the second and third days, plus a couple of glasses of orange juice; after the third day greater latitude may be permitted. The digestive organs have by that time adjusted themselves to the intake of food, and are ready and willing to handle any normal amounts that may be taken. Of course it is far better to induce the patient to eat only wholesome foods — instead of those he formerly indulged in, probably — and in right combinations. Numerous good books on the market deal with these questions, and these should be studied before the fast is broken, so that the right selections may be made.

The above paragraphs cover the main points which should be remembered in breaking a fast, and we may perhaps summarize them very briefly:

1. Do not break the fast until natural hunger returns.

2. Do not continue fasting after it returns.

3. The first two "meals" should consist of a glass of diluted orange juice, sipped and drunk very slowly.

4. The third meals — providing the first solid food — must be very light, eaten slowly and masticated thoroughly.

5. This may consist of any of the various suggested items, according to the likes and preferences of the patient.

6. Only two light meals a day for the first three days.

. After that, greater variety and quantity of food may be allowed — eaten slowly, as before.

8. Care must be taken not to overeat during the first two weeks after breaking the fast. The patient will probably develop a tremendous appetite, after the first day or so; but this must be governed and kept in check, if the best results are to follow.

9. Will power must be exercised in this restraint — as it was during the fast. Emphasize this necessity.

10. Now is a good time to introduce a more sensible diet than the patient formerly indulged in. If this be followed, in moderation, there is no reason why the subject should ever again have to undertake a fast. Years of abuse were required to render a prolonged fast necessary!

AFTER BREAKING THE FAST

"Fasting will not make one disease proof," as Doctor Shelton wisely remarked. "The fast is in vain," said Doctor Tilden, "if the patient returns to his old habits." After the fast is broken, a ravenous appetite frequently develops — as we have said — and this must be kept in check, or unpleasant consequences may follow. The patient may well make himself ill again by over-eating, in which case the benefits derived from the fast are largely negated. Even if this is avoided, a return to the so-called "normal" diet — consisting of three full meals a day — may well result in trouble later on, even though this be some months or years later. If the body is again abused, it will ultimately rebel, necessitating a second or a third fast, in order to normalize it. If due care be taken of the diet, these subsequent periods of abstinence will not be necessitated.

The wisest and simplest plan, surely, is to reform the diet, making it simpler and more wholesome in quality, and more abstemious in quantity. If a little will power be used, this should be easy. The fast has shrunk the stomach, so that it will not crave such large quantities of food, being satisfied with less. Only constant over-eating will again distend it, so that the stomach does not seem satisfied unless this distention is present. In other words, the patient must make himelf sick all over again! But of coure it is quite possible to do this; and the only logical prevention is to cut-down on the food eaten; until a normal physiological balance is maintained. Two meals a day will suffice, and these are all that should be eaten. Fruits should constitute an essential part of the diet. Bearing these simple rules in mind, there is no reason why the patient should not remain in excellent health for years, once he has regained his health through the fast-cure.

CONCLUDING REMARKS

Before a confirmed smoker can break the habit he must first of all really *want* to stop smoking. If he has this sincere desire, breaking the habit is easy. Much the same is true of fasting. The patient must first of all want to get well, and be determined to do so, despite temporary inconveniences, and if he has this "will to be well," he can undertake a fast with a minimum of physical and mental hardship. (Patients who are seriously ill can of course fast with the greatest of ease, since food is usually repugnant to them.)

The first two or three days of the fast are usually the hardest — since the habits of a life-time are being conquered. And there may be brief periods of unpleasantness, from time to time, during its progress. But if the patient keeps steadily in mind the beneficial objectives which may be attained — in consequence of his fast — and force himself through these brief periods, he will be amply rewarded in the long-term benefits he derives from it. These may be noted for weeks, months and even years after the fast has been terminated. If this be borne constantly in mind, a fast may usually be undertaken with relative ease.

The prospective faster must understand the philosophy and physiology of the treatment, realize what is happening and appreciate the meaning of the various symptoms that may arise. In order to gain this preliminary confidence, he should make a study of the literature of the subject, realize what others have found and what he can do also. Fired with this enthusiasm, he can undertake a fast with safety, almost with pleasure. Fasting is usually much easier than generally imagined. Moreover it is really curing him! It is the most powerful and effective remedial agent known to man. This little book is an attempt to prove that fact to the previously uninformed reader. I can only hope that, in this, I have in some degree succeeded.

APPENDIX

The following cases of fasting were for the most part sent to me shortly after the publication of my book, in 1908. Many similar cases have of course been published of late years, and may be found scattered through the literature of the subject, and in journals devoted to health reform. Many of these cases present points of unusual interest, however, for one reason or another, and because of this are included here. The cases follow.

*   *   *   *

The report which follows was in the form of a letter, written me in August, 1913, by Mrs. Maud L. Sharpe, of Chestnut Hill, Mass. She says in part:

Mr. F.—has, I understand, spoken of my fast to you, and I feel that it may interest you to know that I am today on the thirty-fifth day of it — having never dreamed at the start that I could exceed a week at the most!

I started very much weakened after a two weeks' attack of gall-stones, and could hardly stand, being never out of pain; morphine could not quiet me. . . . I gained daily in physical strength and mental vigor and energy, and the elimination has seemed to be indicated by pain in every spot that ever had any trouble! A tumor, diagnosed first thirteen years ago, has disappeared — to sight at least. . . . I have been very happy and full of joy and hope, and I have read all the fasting books, and my own experience is teaching me just where I agree and where not! It is the most vital and interesting of subjects. Your marvelous book, "Vitality, Fasting and Nutrition" has been read eagerly, and I place it among the greatest and most illuminating of books. It is seldom that one can read so many hundred pages and find oneself agreeing with and understand it completely . . .

Today I helped prepare an elaborate 'company' luncheon for out-of-town friends, and sat at the table while it was served, without even wanting water, or having even the slightest desire for the terribly good things they had to eat. . . . I have had no nausea, no faintness, and slept divinely, and am very happy to think that fasting IS a pleasant cure. . . . Thank you for your colossal, helpful work. I wish it were a law for everyone to read it!

*   *   *   *

The following letter was sent me by Mr. H. A. Nouredin Addis, of Long Beach, Calif., in October, 1919:

Mr. J. Austin Shaw has told me that you would like to hear from me in regard to my fasting. There was nothing remarkable about my fast. Everything went on as it should. Fortunately I was able to sleep almost continuously during the first three or four days, thus obviating the unpleasant features of former fasts. Some sixteen or seventeen days elapsed before I experienced any noticeable improvement, but then things began to ameliorate gradually, and I found an actual increase in vitality and strength.

About the beginning of the fifth week I felt so energetic that I began working pretty hard for from one to three hours every day in our vegetable garden. On the afternoon of the forty-fourth day I planted a patch of sweet corn, working hard for several hours.

On the forty-fifth day there was a change. My tongue cleared up, and in the afternoon I felt weak. Yet my color was good and I looked better than usual. My fasting did me an immense amount of good. I think I should add that my fast was a complete one.

Nothing but water passed my lips during those forty-seven days. I began the fast weighing 206 and finished weighing 146. Now I weigh 183, between six and seven weeks after breaking the fast. . . .

*   *   *   *

The following letter from Mr. A. Thommen, Auburn, Calif., was sent me in April, 1912. I quote only those parts of it which refer to fasting:

. . . . It was your book which made it possible for me to undertake a fast which lasted for 49 days. During all that time your practical treatment in each chapter and your common-sense conclusions kept my faith up to the last. Not once did I lose my serene peace of mind in the midst of scoffing, jeering and discouragement. And all the time the absolute certainty of how to start eating again eased my mind and made me assured that no bad effects would follow. . . . My pulse and temperature went to normal as soon as the fast was broken. I feel better than I have in years. I feel more than ever convinced that fasting is the great cure for suffering humanity; my own experience has shown this!

*   *   *   *

Los Angeles, Calif.
February 15, 1911

Dr. Hereward Carrington
Dear Sir:

I take the liberty of writing this letter after reading your book, *Vitality, Fasting and Nutrition,* which has been a revelation to me. Your book was brought to my attention by an article on "Fasting" by Upton Sinclair, which appeared in the February number of the "Cosmopolitan," and which interested me greatly, having been troubled with indigestion for the past ten years, with greater or lesser severity. In this article,

118

he mentions a previous one, on the same subject, in the May number of last year, in which he referred to your publication, together with those of Dr. Dewey, Mr. Macfadden, and others.

My present condition has extended back for a number of years, beginning with a severe attack of heart palpitation, brought on by too many good things at Christmas dinner; and, never having had an attack of this kind before. I thought my last hour had come! My trouble really dates from that time, and if I had only listened to Nature's call, then no doubt my case would not have become chronic, and I should have prevented the misery, irritability and general ill-health of a confirmed dyspeptic. An intimate friend of mine, a physician, did everything in his power to cure me with medicine, and admitted that my nervous temperament counteracted a cure, and finally told me it was just like throwing medicine down a sewer — which condition he himself had brought about by making a sewer of me. The greatest benefit I received was when he placed me on a liquid diet, with hot compresses to the pit of the stomach. I tried to diet myself from time to time; tried homeopathic and osteopathic treatment, without benefit, and finally I was unable to retain food at all. Sometimes I seemed to be continually suffering from too much acid in the stomach, causing food to sour and ferment. As nature seemed to assert itself in such a forcible manner, and as I had no desire for food, I decided to stop eating altogether and to fast.

Having always lived a sedentary life for the past twenty years, practising my profession as an architect, lack of exercise, no doubt, had much to do with my trouble. I am nearly 40 years of age, 5 ft. 6½ in. in height, weight 123 pounds, with clothes on, but physically way below par, and also below normal weight —145 pounds, about.

I was so confident that I should be benefitted, after reading Mr. Sinclair's article, that, without reading-up on the subject or consulting a physician, I started my fast, and, as several symptoms developed during that period which you do not mention in your book, I am sure you will be interested in hearing of them, and possibly can explain them to me, being an authority on the subject.

Before my fast, I had been suffering for about three months with a sort of lump in the throat, which was accompanied by belching of gas, and sometimes food, which the doctor told me was caused by gas and hyperacidity; but which he could relieve in 5 weeks' treatment. This so-called "lump in the throat" continued throughout my fast, and another physician said it was caused by the empty stomach which created a vacuum in the throat. My first doctor put me on a liquid diet, then light food, allowing one cup of coffee with a meal, and when I mentioned Fletcherism ridiculed all such "bosh," as he termed it, as well as the different food cults. Still, he gave me no relief with his 5 weeks' treatment, and was horrified when I mentioned raw fruit, which I seemed to crave since coming to California—the land of fruit and nuts—in search of health.

The following is a brief daily account of my fast:
1st Day. Thursday, January 19, 1910. Weight 123 lbs., with clothes on. Drank cup of hot water for breakfast; glass of malted milk and crackers at noon. Slept 9 hours; worked 7½ hours at office.
2nd Day. Cup of hot beef-tea in morning, with cracker; the same at night. Worked 8 hours. Retired 10 p. m. Took physic to move bowels.

3rd Day. Same as previous day. In evening took egg in beef tea. Took two pills to act on bowels. Slept 9 hours. Drank about 6 glasses of water during the day. Worked 4 hours.

4th Day. Cup of hot water in the morning; cup of beef-tea at noon, with cracker and bread crust. Spent afternoon on beach walking about. There from 12 to 5 p. m. In evening, beef-tea with egg. Slept 9 hours.

5th Day. Total abstinence from food. Drank lots of water. Feeling of great lassitude. Spent evening at Architectural Exhibition; on feet continuously from 9 to 10:30 p. m. Worked 7½ hours. Slept 8 hours. Mind very clear. Still have swallowing sensation or lump in throat.

6th Day. Arose at 7:15 a. m. Felt dizzy on getting up, which wore off after a little. Took cold sponge bath. Took ¾-hour walk at noon. Have a pounding in the left ear or deafness when on my feet. Took low enema in evening. Retired at 11:30 p. m. after having spent evening at theatre. Weight at noon, 117 lbs., with clothes on. Worked 7½ hours.

7th Day. Very dizzy after getting up. Took cold sponge. Pain in back and legs. Felt weak when walking about. Pounding in ear continues. Voice very weak. Very foul breath and coated tongue. Still have lump in throat. Weight at noon 114 lbs. To bed at 9 p. m. Always drink about 3 quarts of water. Worked 7½ hours.

8th Day. Passed restless night, after 3 a. m. Up at 7:30 a. m., feeling dizzy. Cold sponge. Still have lump in throat, and pounding in ear, when walking about. Retired at 9 p. m. Worked 7½ hours. Weight at noon, 113 lbs. Voice very weak, at times. Foul breath. Took low enema.

9th Day. Up at 7:30; felt dizzy and sick at stomach.

121

Pains in kidneys. Voice very weak. Still have pounding in ear and lump in throat, due to gas in stomach. Had to leave office at 4 p. m. Felt better after resting at home. Retired 8 p.m. Pulse 72. Weight 111½ lbs.

10th Day. Up at 7:30 a. m., after a restless night. Felt weak and dizzy on arising. Very foul breath and bad taste in mouth. Pains in legs when walking. Pounding in left ear, when on my feet, and swallowing sensation continues in my throat, annoying me a great deal. Ringing in ears; severe pains in back. Worked 4 hours. Retired 8 p. m.

11th Day. Same as previous one. Very restless night. Drank pint of Appolonaris water, as distilled water seems to gag. Retired 8 p. m.

12th Day. Symptoms same as previous day. Retired at 9 p. m. Weak. Weight, 109½ lbs.

13th Day. Up at 10 a. m. after restless night. Was out of doors all day; *feel stronger.* Took some homeopathic medicine for lump in throat. Retired at 9 p. m. Pulse irregular.

14th Day. Spent another restless night; did not feel so dizzy today when on my feet. Pulse 80 and regular. Broke fast in evening, with glass of grape juice. Lump in throat still annoyed me a good deal. Weight 107 lbs.

15th Day. Up at 9 a. m. Slept well. Had glass of grape juice; juice of one orange at noon; and two in evening. Still have lump in throat. Retired at 9 p. m.

1st Day on Milk Diet. Started drinking ½ pint of milk, warm, at 1 hour intervals. Drank 2 quarts. Walked a good deal. Weight 110 lbs.

2nd Day of Milk Diet. Drinking milk at ¾-hour intervals — ½ pint, warm.

3rd Day Milk Diet. Drinking milk at ½-hour intervals; ½ pint, warm. Juice of orange in morning.

Drink 5 quarts water per day; juice of 2 oranges in evening.

Continuing with milk diet, on the 4th day I weighed 113 lbs.; 5th day, 115 lbs.; 6th day, 116 lbs.; 7th day, same; 8th day, reduced quantity of milk and had first meal at noon, consisting of split pea soup, 2 oatmeal crackers, preserved figs, nuts and raisins, and a glass of milk. In evening had soup and boiled rice. During the entire time on the milk diet, my nerves were very calm and quiet, and I slept well. When I started to eat again, I had trouble with gland on the left side of my neck, near the ear, which would swell and pain as soon as I took the first mouthful of food, and continued through the meal. I had this trouble for about a month before taking the fast, and I hoped that the fast would cure it. I took the milk diet which Mr. Mcfadden recommended, and on this diet gained 9 lbs. in 8 days. As he seems to agree with you as to raw foods, I have tried to use this diet as much as possible, with the addition of two glasses of sumik or clabbered milk. In the evening I take about 3 table-spoonfulls of raisins and about 8 or 10 walnuts. Do you consider that enough food in my case? And what other raw foods would you recommend in my case?

In conclusion, I wish to say that, although not completely cured, I have been greatly benefitted by the fast, and at some future time I will take a finish fast. I have no desire for liquor or smoking, although I had smoked for 20 years. I had quite a time to get your book at the library, as it seemed to be always out, and judging by its condition, they will soon have to get a new volume. It should be in every household, as, I am sure, your future work on diet. Thanking you for taking up so much of your time,

Sincerely yours,
ALFRED KUHN.

San Francisco, Calif.
June 7, 1910.

Dr. Hereward Carrington

Dear Sir:

Your letter of May 29th at hand. It gives me pleasure to confirm the report which you have read in regard to my fasting experience. I am enclosing a copy of my record for the eight days of my fast.

I am pleased to state that the effects of the fast were so beneficial that I have been instrumental in inducing a number of my friends to undergo the same treatment. Being a physician myself, I have been able to benefit quite a number of people in this way.

Trusting this information may be of use to you. I am,

Yours sincerely,
CLARENCE E. EDWARDS.

RECORD OF FAST

Beginning: Weight 197 pounds. Waist measure 46 inches. Height 5 ft. 6 in. Chronic kidney trouble. Periodical headaches, sometimes lasting 3 or 4 days. Easily tired. Dragging feeling after day's work. Sleep broken and restless. Abnormal appetite. Disinclination to physical exercise. Touches of articular rheumatism in fingers.

First Day. Weight 194½ lbs. No change in conditions. Drank two pints of water on arising, one with juice of half a lemon in it, the other clear. Drank one pint of hot water in evening. Drank about two pints of cold water during the day. Drank one pint of Shasta water before retiring. Walked 5 miles during the day. No appreciable hunger.

Second Day. Weight 192 lbs. Drank water as on first day. Slight headache in morning, which passed off before noon. Slightly hungry, but surprised that I have no excessive craving for food. Feel lighter, and mind is clearer than usual. Rest broken more than usual last night, owing to excessive activity of kidneys. No perceptible change in condition other than those noted. Stayed in the house all day, sleep and reading.

Third Day. Weight 189½ lbs. Slight headache all day. Drank hot and cold water, same as on previous days. Slept soundly during the night with little interruption. Feel weakness about knees. Walked 4 miles. No hunger at all.

Fourth Day. Weight 188 lbs. Same water as on previous days. Feel light and active, with desire for exercise. Mind clear and active. Rested well last night. No ache or pain. Walked 5 miles during the day.

Fifth Day. Bad headaches. Extreme lassitude. Weight 186½ lbs. Weak knees. Dragged through the day and got home almost exhausted. As I had been a confirmed coffee drinker for more than 40 years, I attributed my condition to the sudden breaking-off of this habit, and took a cup. I at once felt better. I decided that if weakness and lassitude continued in the morning I would break fast. Slept well during the night. Walked 3 miles. Drank hot and cold water as usual.

Sixth Day. Weight 186½ lbs. Surprised at there being no loss of weight. Drank a cup of coffee in the morning, in addition to the usual hot water. Felt fine all day. No ache or pain, and mind clear and active. Great desire for exercise. Walked 9 miles. Slept well at night. Kidney trouble greatly improved.

Seventh Day. Weight 186½ lbs. No loss in weight in past 2 days. Feel extraordinarily well and active, both physically and mentally. Walked 5 miles. No ache or pain anywhere. Physical appearance greatly improved. Waist measure 41 inches.

Eighth Day. Weight 185 lbs. Strong and active. Feel like taking a great amount of physical exercise. Mentally clear and active. During all week, I have continued regular work without intermission. Go home in evening now bright and fresh, even on days of excessive work. Improvement of condition so marked that I shall continue fasting further. . . .

(No further reports received. H.C.)

* * * *

Here follow four letters, representing four different cases, which were written me by men who had undertaken the fast, and were quite "unsolicited testimonials" in the best sense of the word. They all present certain points of interest, which are well brought out in the accounts themselves—

Malta, Sliema
26 April, 1911.

Dr. Hereward Carrington
Dear Sir:

I have just finished a fast of forty days, and my wife one of thirty-three, only on water. If you think the experience of any interest to you, I shall be glad to forward you any information you desire about it. Your admirable work, published by Rebman and Co., has been our reliable guide during our long fast. There are several interesting things to add to your experience, and some which do not altogether agree with it; but it would take much time to communicate all this by correspondence. I am at present preparing my book on fasting in Italian, which will contain all my present experience about the subject, and as soon as published I shall be very pleased to send you a copy. It was your book which determined my wife and myself to undergo the miraculous cure of fasting. I am enclosing a photo, taken on the 40th day of my fast; also one taken before I began my fast.* You will note the difference! With many hearty and sincere thanks for your kindness, believe me,

With best regards,

Sincerely yours,

A. LEVANZIN, B.A.

*   *   *   *

La Junta, Colo.
March 28, 1911.

Dr. Hereward Carrington
Dear Sir:

I read your "Vitality, Fasting and Nutrition" at the Public Library, in Hot Springs, Ark., where I had gone, with a swelling in my groin. . . . I first of all took a fast of eight days, breaking it on the ninth; but later took a fast of 27 days, keeping an account of this. I had to go to the hospital for treatment for another matter, however; and the doctor told me that if I did not eat something by 7 p. m., he would have me placed in an insane asylum, that I was starving to death, etc. So I had to break my fast, which I did on hot milk. . . . I am a new man. I awake and get out of bed at daylight — a thing I have not done for years, and it's a pleasure when I breathe — the air seems to go right down to my toes. I want to take a complete fast some time. I am sorry I had to break this fast at the end of 27 days, and think I am a coward for letting that doctor scare me with the insane asylum. . . . Your

---

*Mr. Levanzin afterward took a 31-day experimental fast in Boston, under the supervision of the Carnegie Nutrition Laboratories: see their voluminous reports "A Study of Prolonged Fasting," and "Inanition and Metabolism".

book has done a world of good, and I am not slow in its praise.

Very respectfully,
CLAUSON JONES.

*   *   *   *

September 13, 1910.

Rebman Co., New York
Gentlemen:

I have just finished Hereward Carrington's *Vitality, Fasting and Nutrition,* and have finished an 11-day fast, with not one bad symptom. I have gone right ahead with the same routine as before, without any inconvenience, while my system has been toned-up to a point it has not known for years. I am 62 years old; I shall carry the fast through to the proper termination. It would be absolutely impossible to express my gratitude and appreciation, and the book has been a fascinating revelation to me from beginning to end. . . . I would appreciate it very much if you would send me the latest and best work on the value of food for nutrition; what I have seen so far do not measure-up, in their line, to "V. F. and N.," and I thought there might be something later and better.

Yours truly,
ED. H. JOHNSON

*   *   *   *

March 5, 1910.

Dr. Hereward Carrington
Dear Sir:

I have looked you up, read and re-read your masterly work "Vitality and Fasting," and am convinced you are "on the level,'" and deserve the intense and eternal gratitude of every friend of mankind. I note you have given Trall, Graham, Nicols, Page, Walter, Dewey, etc., due and full credit, for which I personally thank you. You have got down to "bed rock" as no other living or dead author ever has, I firmly believe. Anthro-therapy, in the light of your efforts, is to my mind an exact science, a positive art. I personally know or did know Mrs. Eddy, Dr. Walter, Drayton, Page, Kellogg, Purinton, etc.

Now as to my fast, I can add but one interesting feature, which I am willing to repeat. I had "normal hunger" on the 4th day and, of course, every day thereafter. I lost about 20-22 pounds. I regained them all — good solid fighting weight, on boiled potatoes — no salt — just boiled potatoes, and water.

Pardon my long delay.

May you live a happy, healthy and useful life.

Most respectfully,

CHARLES D. HAMILTON

*   *   *   *

In the following case I have unfortunately lost the early correspondence; but the gist of it was that my present correspondent's father was seriously ill, and wished to undertake a fast, and asked me where he could go to take it. I recommended the Macfadden Sanitarium and received, some days later, the following letter, saying that the father had died before his removal to the Sanitarium had been been possible. Meanwhile, however, the son commenced a fast, and the results of this are detailed below:

May 28, 1910.

Dr. Hereward Carrington:
Dear Sir:

Before receiving your letter, my father passed away, so that I could not have him sent to the Macfadden Sanitorium, as you suggested. I had, however, completed the reading of your very valuable work, and began with one meal a day on April 10th, eating my last meal April 13th. On Thursday, the 14th, at the usual hour for the one meal, I had an intense craving for food, which caused bile in the stomach to such an extent that it nauseated me. This only lasted a few minutes, when, after vomiting, all desire for food left me and did not return. The bowels also moved at that time, and again naturally in the mornings on the 18th and 23rd, and 27th and 30th. I tried to let nature have its course, and did not use the enema until May 9th, when I used it and for the next two days, partly in accordance with your suggestion; but I found that I secured better results by elevating the hips on a padded box and lying on the back for the third injection. I was at my office, and did my usual work up to May 10th, through the 26th day of my fast, but being quite weak on that day, I stayed at home and continued to do so for one week; *i.e.*, until 4 days after I had broken the fast, which was May 11th, at 11 p. m., by eating just the juice of an orange and about $\frac{1}{4}$ the juice of a grapefruit. My tongue had not yet cleared and I had no natural hunger, but business matters were coming up which demanded my attention, and I was compelled to break the fast against my will, before deriving the full benefit. I did secure great benefit, however, entirely freeing myself from chronic nasal catarrh, and other minor troubles. My skin is like a baby's, and even my hair is thicker and improved in quality.

Thanking you for the great benefit I have derived from your work, I remain,

Yours for a higher life,

JUDSON M. PERRY

Mr. W. E. Whyte, of London, England, wrote me in July, 1913, that he had just completed, most successfully, a fast of fifty-six days. This was undertaken under the care of Dr. Rabagliati, who intended to publish an account of it later. (If this account was ever published, I regret that I failed to see it).

Writing me in October, 1920, Dr. Edward O. Johnstone, of Buffalo, New York, said:

"Relative to my fast . . . I sent a brief account of this to "Physical Culture" magazine, which appeared in the August issue of 1912 or 1914 — I just cannot recall which year. The article bore the assumed name of Terrae Filius. . . . The shortest fast I ever undertook was four days and the longest 32 days. I have fasted six different times. . . . I am a thorough believer in fasting and am convinced that if fasting will not cure, then the patient had better prepare for a celestial harp! Your book has taught me much and I thank you. . . ."

*   *   *   *

In the following case, the early correspondence is again lost, but, as I recollect it, the patient wrote to me for advice, stating that he suffered from "worms," and I recommended a fast, followed by a strictly fruitarian diet. Some weeks later, I again wrote the patient, asking him how his fast had progressed, and received the following letter in reply:

January 21, 1909

Dr. Hereward Carrington:
Dear Sir:

With regard to your letter of the 6th instant, in reply to mine re the question of worms during fasting, in which you ask me to inform you how the fast terminated, I may say that I maintained a fast for 26 days.

What I mistook for worms was nothing but strings of mucus from the colon; I had a microscopic test made. My experience appears to be somewhat contradictory to the statements made in your work, in the following respects: My object in fasting was that I had for years abused my stomach by eating, and suffered always intense weakness and possessed even greater hunger after the ingestion of a meal than before, etc. Also, I had suffered from chronic discharges from the nose, and although I took a great deal of treatment for this, I thought that probably the improved condition of the blood under the fast would replace this diseased tissue. On or about the 4th day of the fast, my tongue had a light coating, and my breath was not pleasant. This continued, or became worse until the 15th day, when my breath became normal, the tongue partially cleared, the odor previously noticed from the skin had stopped, and the pink color appeared under the finger nails; but the water, after taking an enema, continued still to be returned "dark," with strings of mucus. The elimination of feces had stopped. My pulse was still what it had been all along, since starting the fast, 54 to 70, and my temperature the same, being anywhere from 96.8° to 98.0°. My weight at the beginning of the fast was 150 lbs., and at its conclusion 127 lbs., but as I was still getting the usual amount of discharge of mucus from my nose and throat, I decided that the fast was in no wise complete, especially as hunger had not yet returned. I still continued, and, apart from the continued loss of weight and intense weakness, conditions did not change. I had little desire for water, and some days drank only about one-half a pint. On one day, I drank none, and I noticed a swelling of the tongue and a tightness of the throat. The doctors here advised me to break the fast, as they stated the coating on the tongue was not a pathological one, and therefore could not be indicative of the condition of the alimentary canal. I did not wish to break the fast, so continued until the 26th day, and, no change appearing, I broke the fast. I lost 34 lbs. during the 25 days. I have the idea in my head to undergo another fast when summer comes, as winter is no time for fasting in a cold climate for various reasons. During the fast, I had my blood pressure taken every 5 days, a blood test taken every 5 days, and my urine examined and measured every 5 days, and, strange to say, on the 15th day, these conditions were nearer normal than when I broke the fast 11 days later,* being on the 15th day:

Red Corpuscles	7,095,200
Lcyts.	6,000
Hgbln.	100%
Blood Pressure	123

I should like your opinion as to whether I should have continued my fast until the removal of the diseased membrane of the nose. The condition at present is the same as ever. My fast was broken Jan. 1, and at present I have regained 24 lbs. of my lost weight.

I am,

Sincerely yours,

GILBERT THOMSON

*   *   *   *

In the case which follows, the fasts were of especial interest, because of the age of both patients. Moreover, it will be seen that great benefit can be derived

*To my mind, this seems natural enough, since the fast ended really at this time, and starvation began on that day - a very different thing. The return of natural hunger on the 15th day clearly indicated that the fast should have been broken then; and a careful course of dieting would doubtless have removed the remainder of the trouble, in time. -H.C.

from a strict fast, on occasion, even if the previous habits of life and dietetic habits have been extremely abstemious. Accompanying this letter was a newspaper clipping — giving an account of the fast; and I have copied one or two paragraphs from this, which present points of some interest, not brought out in the following letter—

Dear Dr. Carrington:

I have read your book, *Vitality, Fasting and Nutrition* aloud to my wife with more interest than any other book I have ever read on hygiene, and I have read a great many. Yours is the only one that does not leave out some important health factor. You have condensed the cream of libraries and have got in all the chief factors. And I advise everybody, if necessary, to pawn their watch and buy one of your books. I have already ordered five for friends. I have read most of the writers you quote, and have been personally acquainted with Drs. Lewis, Emmet Densmore, Otto Carque, James C. Jackson, Alice B. Stockham, and others. Reinhold, Jackson, Kuhne, and others have written good books on health, but they all lack some essential factor. Take Dr. Jamison, for instance. I have sold a good many of his "Intestinal Ills," and "Intestinal Irrigation" to people seeking advice from me. But he is in a rut, and can see but one important factor. I have also sold a great many of C. C. Haskell's books. But he fails to see the importance of Jamison's chief factor. But you seem to have made an exhaustive study of the subject, and have got in all the chief factors. And I for one wish to congratulate you.

I found no new ideas in your book except regarding the derivation of our heat and energy. Your ideas on this subject are certainly new and interesting, and your arguments seem very logical. But, if your ideas are correct, we will have to modify our diet very greatly, it seems to me. Our object in eating is to supply broken down tissue wholly. The question arises: What elements are required to supply broken down tissue, and in what proportion? An egg to hatch a perfect bird must contain albumen, fat and certain salts. The ox or horse finds sufficient of these three things in grass to supply their tissues, when in a natural state. But when put to work by man, extra grains, containing more protein, are required to supply the waste. So probably man in a natural state could repair all bodily waste from raw fruits, (an ox will grow fat on pears and sweet apples), but when working will he not need a certain amount of nuts or legumes? I infer from something I read in your book that you are preparing a work on foods. Am I correct? I hope so. It is very important that such a book should be published in the light of your new ideas regarding the true use of food.*

As to our "conquest fast," we are more convinced than ever that fasting is the panacea for about all the ills to which flesh is heir. But we found a great deal of difficulty in drinking much water while we were fasting. Perhaps our daily, copious enemas aided in this direction. Still, we felt the need for some water in the stomach to obtain the most pleasant results. I usually had to put a few drops of fruit juice (unfermented grape) in the water in order to drink it without decided repugnance.

I have made a study of hygiene for over 50 years and am getting new ideas every little while. My wife has eaten but one meal a day for over ten years. I had

*"The Natural Food of Man," subsequently published (1912).
-H.C.

eaten but one meal a day this year until I began this fast. But I think I will resume my life-long habit of two meals a day; 8:30 a. m., and 4:30 p. m., being careful to have but one article or kind of food at each meal. I have taken a cabinet bath every other morning on rising, followed by a cold plunge, for 30 years. I rub my body with olive oil after each bath. We live in a house of my wife's own designing and building. The primary object was light and fresh air. We sleep upstairs. And there are no glass windows on that floor. . . . About sunrise and sundown daily I take a three-mile walk, walking over 2,000 miles each year. I have been doing this for nearly six years. . . .

Yours for progress,

D. EDSON SMITH

Extract from a Newspaper Cutting *re* this case—

REMARKABLE FEATS OF FASTING BY AGED COUPLE

Mr. and Mrs. D. Edson Smith, each nearly seventy years of age, fasted thirty-seven and thirty-one days respectively, with highly beneficial results. Mr. Smith declares his belief that pure air, cleanliness and proper diet will surely prevent and cure all bodily ills. . . .

- - - - - -

After eating one meal, chiefly of fruit, every other day for a month, Mrs. Smith had so reduced her flesh that she weighed but 96 pounds. She then, on the last day of June, began a complete fast, taking only distilled water. All hunger left her on the third day, and did not return till after thirty-one days and four hours, when a strong desire for food came, which was gratified, first with orange juice, and then with a little parched sweet corn-meal gruel. For several days the diet was chiefly stewed, or raw, tomatoes and stewed onions and rice.

The benefits accruing from this fast were most wonderful. At the beginning of the fast, her legs and feet seemed like wooden ones. No feeling in them. . . . The feeling of childhood days was restored. An exhausted stomach seems fully restored. A central difficulty of forty years' standing was removed. The eyesight is very greatly improved. The general tone is better than in years. . . .

*   *   *   *

The following case-record was sent me some years ago, quite spontaneously. Only essential extracts are quoted, as the record itself is lengthy, and full of disquisitional material. Mr. Kruse had taken several fasts before, including one of thirty-one days — as the record indicates. The following fast lasted 25 days. His Diary reads in part:

First Day - January 26th, 1933.

Started my fast in a new, unique and involuntary manner — this time, although I had planned to fast in the near future.

It happened aboard ship, after leaving Jacksonville, Fla., bound for New York. At Jacksonville I happened to weigh myself, weighing 146 pounds; allowing eight pounds for my clothes, leaves me 138 pounds in the nude, which has been my average weight for life.

Travelling down the St. John's river in the evening hours of January 25th, I ate a hearty dinner, but soon afterwards we ran into a rough ocean; the ship was rolling from side to side all throughout the night, and most of the passengers became sea-sick, including myself — a one time sailor. Every bit of food that had been eaten the night before was promptly vomited, and, as the sea got rougher and rougher, during the following first day of our journey out of Jacksonville, I got sicker and sicker. All thoughts of food and eating were banished! It was the most miserable night and day of my life.

Second Day.

Miserable as was the first day of my fast and journey, the second day was far worse. Around Cape Hatteras, the waves hit the ship from all sides, so that it was not only rolling, but pitching as well. The screws of the big liner were much out of the water, and jerking as if the ship would break. . . .

We arrived six hours late in New York. I felt very spent and chilly, after getting out of my berth, and long before I went ashore I had resolved to continue fasting. . . .

Third Day.

I was quite busy all day. Drank two bottles of "water," which purged me clean within an hour. (I had had a bowel movement each day before). Weighed exactly 140 pounds. . . .

Fourth Day.

Have less headache than I had before. My stomach hurts me much at times, but not at all times. Drank about two quarts of water. Tongue is coated, but not badly.

Fifth Day.

Wrote letters and walked much. Drank water often, but not in great amounts at a time. I dread the days in which there is nothing to do. To pass away the time while fasting is sometimes a problem; so I planned to keep busy and active throughout. Weight 138 pounds.

Sixth Day.

Pulse somewhat slow and irregular, but with an occasional sense of throbbing. Tired in evening and went to bed early.

Seventh Day.

Had my best night. Slept more and rested comfortably. Weight 136 pounds.

Eighth Day.

Had a good night again. Felt a pleasant "itching" sensation in the stomach during the fore-noon. It must be getting better!

Ninth Day.

Tongue badly coated. Weight 134 pounds.

Tenth Day.

No enemas thus far. Weight 133 pounds.

Eleventh Day.

Sunday. To church and a walk. Rested later.

Twelfth Day.

Every time that I have fasted, I can honestly say that I have greatly benefitted by it. The days following a fast are among the happiest in my life, and the most elated. It was as though something permeated my whole being, which I cannot find words to explain.

Thirteenth Day.

Nothing special to report. Feel well. Took a long walk.

Fourteenth Day.

Had a bowel movement in the early morning! Tongue still much coated. Weight 129 pounds; loss about a pound a day.

Fifteenth Day.

Another bowel movement! Drank hot instead of cold water, as the weather is cold.

Sixteenth Day.

My tongue seems to be clearing a bit at the tip.

Walked forty blocks in the bitter cold which, in the end, did me a lot of good. (I walked every day in the fresh air.)

Seventeenth Day.

Weight 126 pounds - a loss of 20 pounds in 17 days.

Eighteenth Day.

I am positive that 'the worst is over,' and that after this it will be much easier to fast. Much writing.

Nineteenth Day.

I find that I am breathing much more freely. No longer any protruding abdomen! Pains in the stomach almost entirely gone.

Twentieth Day.

Tongue still coated, but not so badly. Felt well otherwise.

Twenty-first Day.

· My teeth, the whites of my eyes, the moons on my finger-nails are all getting whiter. My skin is getting to feel as soft as a baby's yet is hardier. The luster of my hair is improving. My eyes are stronger. These are all good signs of improvement.

Twenty-second Day.

I am getting thinner, but there are no wrinkles on my face or elswhere. Not losing much weight; 124 pounds today.

Twenty-third Day.

Not much new to report. Think I shall break my fast next Sunday, after church.

Twenty-fourth Day.

Lost only three pounds this past week.

Twenty-fifth Day.

Last day of fasting . . . And so I consider this Record finished!

JOHN CARL KRUSE

The following is a brief list of cases which have been cured by fasting — notices of which have come to me chiefly through the newspapers and similar sources. As I have no details in most of these instances, I merely summarize them. At least four of them are thoroughly authentic, however, as I happen to know the subjects who underwent the fast. (A very instructive list of cases cured by this method of treatment is to be found in Mr. Upton Sinclair's book. *The Fasting Cure.*)

Mrs. Harriet M. Closz, of Webster City, Iowa, fasted for forty-five days, completely curing herself of "rheumatism," reported at the time in the New York *Times.*

Mr. Edmund R. Taylor, of Cold Run, Ohio, fasted for thirty days for weight-reduction and general health improvement. He continued his activities as a missionary throughout the fast.

Mr. Christ Cortensen, of St. Paul, Minn., fasted for fifty-three days, to a most successful conclusion. (A Case Reported in "The Liberator," August, 1906, p. 115).

Mr. Clifford N. Mackwell, of Newark, N. J., wrote me in 1921 that he had just completed a thirty-five day fast, and speaks of "the exaltation and clarity of mind" which he experienced as a result of it. (This is noted by nearly all fasting patients).

In a letter written in March, 1911, Mr. Alanson Jones, of La Junta, Colo., advised me that he had just completed most successfully, a twenty-seven day fast, and that he contemplated undertaking another one in the near future. (I heard indirectly that he was killed shortly afterwards).

Roland Mueller, engineer, fasted 57 days, for stomach trouble and partial deafness, caused by chronic

,catarrh. Completely cured both. Weight reduced from 148 lbs. to 97½lbs. Broke his fast on fruit. Took olive oil with advantage during the last days of his fast.

Charles Spencer, artist, fasted 40 days, working throughout that period. He only broke his fast when natural hunger returned; "so," he said, "I agree with Hereward Carrington's maxim that the fast should only be ended when normal hunger returns."

Eskholme Wade, of Molesley, Surrey, England, fasted 30 days, for experimental purposes. He ran and walked 30 miles every day. Is a fruitarian the rest of the time.

Mrs. John Dietz, of Winter, Wis., fasted 56 days, curing herself of chronic appendicitis. She lost 59 pounds in weight, all of which was regained after the fast was broken.

Dr. S. M. Stauffer, of Pittsburg, fasted 28 days into perfect health. He cured a debilitated and generally run-down condition by this fast.

George Chapman, of New York, fasted 40 days. Mr. Chapman was known to my friend Maurice V. Samuels, and was interviewed for me by him.

O. E. Eades, of Wanganui, New Zealand, fasted 72 hours, thereby curing a case of piles of some weeks standing.

Dr. Gustav A. Gayer, of New York, well known to me, fasted 30 days to demonstrate "the power of mind over body." He was watched throughout by several physicians, and reports of his case were published daily in the New York papers, and signed by the physicians in attendance. An examination of his blood on the 30th day showed the usual number of red blood corpuscles, and no signs of deterioration. (See *Encyclop. Phys. Cult.*, III., pp. 1319-1322).

Richard Fausel fasted 90 days, losing over 70 pounds. This is one of the longest fasts on record. The subject (foolishly) entered a wrestling contest on the 49th day of his fast! (For details of this remarkable case, see the "Encyclopaedia of Physical Culture," Vol. III, pp 1327-28 and 1362-64).

Many similar cases may be found in Upton Sinclair's "*The Fasting Cure*," and in the literature of the subject. However, the above will probably prove enough for all practical purposes — illustrative of the beneficial results to be obtained from fasting.

BIBLIOGRAPHY

The Bibliography on Fasting which follows does not pretend to be in any way complete; it covers, however, the most important books and articles which I have been enabled to find dealing with *therapeutic* fasting. Such general topics as inanition, starvation, hibernation, etc., may be found listed in Prof. Morgulis's work *Fasting and Undernutrition*, covering some 86 pages. *Books* are in italics. Many articles on fasting have appeared in the pages of "Physical Culture," "The Stuffed Club," "The Hygienic Review," etc., and references may be found scattered throughout books dealing with Nature Cure, Dietetics and general hygiene. Those herein listed deal for the most part almost wholly or exclusively with the subject.

—H. C.

Allen, F. N. Control of experimental diabetes by fasting and total dietary restriction. J. Exp. Med., 31, 575-86. (1920)

Allen, G. D. The rate of oxygen consumption during starvation etc. Amer. J. Physiol., 49, 420-73 1919)

Ash, J. E. The blood in inanition. Arch. Inter. Med., 14, 8-32.

Austin, Major Reynold. *Direct Paths to Health.* (1922)

Barrows, W. The effect of inanition on the structure of the nerve cells. Am. J. Physiol., 1, 14 (1898)

Bassler, A. The Fasting Cure Answered. Month. Cycl. and Med. Bull., 4, 332-44 (1911)

Bean, C. H. Starvation and Mental Development. Psychol. Clin., 3, 78-85 (1908)

Benedict, F. Gano. *The Influence of Inanition on Metabolism.* (1907)

Benedict, F. Gano. *A Study of Prolonged Fasting.* (1915)

Benedict, F. G. & Dufendorf, A. . The analysis of urine in a starving woman. Am. J. Physiol., 18, 362-76. (1907)

Bennett, Sanford. *Old Age: Its Cause and Prevention.* (1921)

Carlson, A. J. *The Control of Hunger in Health and Disease.* (1916)

Carlson, A. J. Hunger, appetite and gastric juice secretion in man during prolonged fasting. Am. J. Physiol., 45, 120-46. (1918)

Carlson, A. J. & Hoelzel, F. *Nutrition, Senescence and Rejuvenescence.* (1951)

Carrington, Hereward. *Vitality, Fasting and Nutrition.* (1908)

Carrington, Hereward. *Death Deferred.* (1912)

Carrington, Hereward. *Fasting for Health.* (LBB): (1928)

Cathcart, E. P. Metabolism during starvation. J. Physiol., 35, 27-32; 500-510. (1907)

Chittenden, R. H. *Physiological Economy in Nutrition.* (1904)

Chittenden, R. H. *The Nutrition of Man.* (1907)

Cornaro, Louis. *The Temperate Life.* (Ed. 1903, entitled "The Art of Living Long.")

Crichton-Browne, Sir James. *Parcimony in Nutrition.* (1909)

Curran, W. The Pathology of Starvation. Med. Press & Circ., Lond., 29, 210-229. (1880)

Curtis, Dr. A Study of blood during a prolonged fast. Proc. Am. As. Adv. Sci., 30, 95-105. (1881)

DeVries, Arnold. *Therapeutic Fasting.* (1949)

145

Densmore, Dr. Emmet. *How Nature Cures.* (1903)

Dewey, E. H. *The True Science of Living.* (1894)

Dewey, E. H. *A New Era for Women.* (1896)

Dewey, E. H. *Chronic Alcoholism.* (1899)

Dewey, E. H. *The No-Breakfast Plan and the Fasting Cure.* (1900)

Dewey, E. H. *Experiences of the No-Breakfast Plan and the Fasting Cure.* (1902)

Eales, Irving J. *Healthology.* (1907)

Ehret, Arnold. *Rational Fasting.* (1920)

Eyre, Sir James *The Stomach, and its Difficulties.* (1869)

Fisher, J. The Effect of Diet on Endurance. (1918)

Fletcher, Horace. The New Glutton or Epicure. (1896)

Fletcher, Horace. The A-B-Z of Our Own Nutrition. (1903)

Foldes, E. A. A new Approach to Dietetic Therapy. (1933)

Frazier, B. C. Prolonged Starvation. Louisville Med. J., 15, 147-54. (1908)

Gandhi, M. K. *Ethics of Fasting.* (1949)

Gordon, Dr. A Prolonged Fast. Montreal Med. J., 36, 482. (1907)

Graham, Sylvester. *The Science of Human Life.* (1843)

Guelpa, Dr. S. *Auto-Intoxication and Disintoxication.* (1910)

Guelpa, Dr. S. Starvation and Purgation in the Relief of Disease. Brit. Med. J., 2, 1050. (1910)

Hammond, W. A. *Fasting Girls.* (1879)

Hanish, Dr. O. *How to Fast.* (N.D.)

Haskell, Charles C. *Perfect Health* **(1901)**

Hay, Wm. H., *Health via Diet.* (1923)

Hay, Mm. H. *A New Health Era.* (1933)

Hazzard, L. B. *Fasting for the Cure of Disease.* (1908)

Hill & Eckman. *The Starvation Treatment of Diabetes.* (1915)

Hoelzel, Fred K. *Fasting, Water and Salt.* (1935)

Hoffman, Dr. *Description of the Magnificent Results Obtained Through Fasting for All Diseases.* (17th. Cent.)

Hoover, Dr. A Study of Metabolism during fasting in hypnotic sleep. J. Exp. Med., 2, 405-11. (1879)

Howe, P. E. & Hawk, P. B. Nitrogen partition and physiological resistance as influenced by repeated fasting. J. Am. Chem. Soc., 33, 215-54. (1910)

Howe, P. E. & Hawk, P. B. On the differential leucocyte count during prolonged fasting. Am. J. Physiol., 30, 174-81. (1912)

Howe, Mattill & Hawk. The influence of an excessive water ingestion on a dog after a prolonged fast. J. Biol. Chem., 10, 417-32. (1911)

Howe, Mattill & Hawk. Distribution of Nitrogen during a fast of one hundred and seventeen days. J. Biol. Chem., 11, 103-27. (1912)

Howe & Hawk. A metabolism study on a fasting man. Proc. Am. Soc. Biol. Chem., 31. (1912)

Jackson, C. M. *Inanition and Malnutrition.* (1925)

Jennings, Isaac. *The Tree of Life.* (1867)

Jennings, Isaac. *Medical Reform.* (1847)

Jennings, Isaac. *Philosophy of Human Life.* (1852)

Jesse, Henry. *The Exceeding Riches of Grace Advanced, by the Spirit of Grace, in an Empty-Nothong Creature, viz. Sarah Wright.* (1647)

Jordon, Edwin O. *Food Poisoning.* (1917)

Kagan, J. Blood and Blood pressure of fasting animals. Diss. St. Petersburg. (1884)

Keith, Dr. George S. *A Plea for a Simpler Life.* (1903)

Keith, Dr. George S. *Fads of an Old Physician.* (1904)

Kellogg, J. H. The Fasting Cure. Good Health, 40, 1-4. (1905)

Kip, Rev. William. *The Lenten Fast.* (1843)

Kiinde, M. M. The After-Effects of Prolonged Fasting on the Basal Metabolic rate. J. Metab. Res., 3,399. (1923)

Langfeld, H. S. On the psychophysiology of a prolonged fast. Psych. Monographs, 16, No. 5. (1914)

MacFadden, B. & Oswald, Felix. *Fasting, Hydropathy and Exercise.* (1904)

MacFadden, Bernarr. *Fasting for Health.* (1923)

MacFadden, B. Fasting, Ency. Phys. Cult., 3, 1203-1396.

Mapes, C. Fasting Int. Clin. Phil., 3, 100-16. (1911)

Mayer, Adolf. Fasting Cures: Wonder Cures. (?)

McCoy, Frank. *The Fast Way to Health.* (1923)

Mapes, J. H. A Fast of 55 Days. Med. Brief., 32, 905. (1904)

McCollum, Simmons, Shipley & Park. The effects of starvation on the healing of rickets. Bull. Johns Hopkins Hosp., 33, 31-33. (1922)

Medvedjeo, J. On Fasting. St. Petersburg. (1882)

Meltzer, S., & Norris, Ch. On the influence of fasting upon the bacteriological action of the blood. J. Exp. Med., 4, 131-35. (1899)

Meyers, A. W. Some morphological effects of prolonged inanition. J. Med. Res., 36, 51-77. (1917)

Morgulis, Serg. *Fasting and Undernutrition.* (1923)

Morgulis, S. The influence of protracted and intermittent fasting upon growth. Am. Naturalist, 477-87. (1913)

Morgulis, Howe & Hawk. Studies of tissues of fasting animals. Biol. Bull., 28, 397-406. (1915)

Morgulis, S. Contributions to the physiology of regeneration. J. Exp. Zool., 7, 595-642. (1909)

Mottram, V. H. Fatty infiltration of the liver in hunger. J. Phys., 38, 281-313. (1909)

Myers, V. C. & Fine, M. S. The influence of starvation upon the creatine content of muscle. J. Biol. Chem., 15, 283-304. (1913)

Nichols, T. L. *The Diet Cure.* (1881)

Okazaki, S. Inanition and the cerebral cortex. Jap. Med. World, 10, 225-26. (1920)

Oldfield, Josiah. *Fasting for Health and Life.* (1924)

Oswald, Felix. *Physical Education.* (1882)

Oswald, Felix. *Nature's Household Remedies.* (1885)

Page, L. C. *The Natural Cure.* (1883)

Paton, N. D. & Stockman, R. Observations on the metabolism of a fasting man. Royal Soc. Edin., 4, 3. (1889)

Penny, F. Notes on a thirty day's fast. Brit. Med. Jo., 1, 1414-16. (1909)

Pottinger, F. M. & Simonsen, D. G. Deficient calcification produced by diet. Trans. Am. Thera. Soc., 39. (1939)

Price, A. W. *Nutrition and Physical Degeneration.* (1939)

Purinton, E. E. *The Philosophy of Fasting.* (1906)

Pyaskovski, N. Fasting from a physiological and hygienic point of view. Sputnik Zdorow., 5, 130-33. (1903)

Rabagliati, A. *Air, Food and Exercises.* (1904)

Rabagliati, A. *Aphorisms, Definitions, Reflections and Paradoxes.* (1901)

Rabagliati, A. *Food and its Relation to Energy and Heat.* (1907)

Rabagliati, A. *Conversations with Women.* (1910)

Rabagliati, A. *A New Theory of Energy.* (Introduction to Carrington's *Vitality, Fasting and Nutrition*). (1908)

Sands, N. J. Prolonged fasting as a factor in the treatment of acute disease, etc. N. Y. State J. Med., 4, 55. (1904)

Seaton, Julia. *Regeneration Through Fasting.* (1929)

Shaw, J. Austin. *The Best Thing in the World.* (1905)

Shelton, Herbert M. *The Hygienic System* (Vols. 3, 7, etc.)

Shew, Dr. Joel. *The Hydropathic Family Physician.* (1850)

Sinclair, Upton. *The Fasting Cure.* (1911)

Smith, Ellen G. *The Art of Living.* (1902)

Stern, Heinrich. *Fasting and Undernutrition in the Treatment of Diabetes.* (1916)

Szekely, Edmund B. *The Therapeutics of Fasting.* (1942)

Szekely, E. B. *Fasting and Grape Cure.* (1950)

Talbot, Dr. *Deaths from Starvation,* etc. Lond., 1903. (Gov. Rept.)

Tilden, J. H. *Toxemia Explained.* (1926)

Tilden, J. H. *Criticisms of the Practice of Medicine.* (1909)

Trall, R. T. *Hydropathic Encyclopedia.* (1850). (Also other books of Dr. Trall's).

Twain, Mark. *The Man that Corrupted Hadleyburg,* etc. (1900). (Contains two articles on fasting).

Walter, Robert. *Vital Science.* (1899)

Walter, Robert. *The Exact Science of Health.* (1903)

Walter, Robert. *The New Science of Living.* (1907)

Weger, George S. *The Genesis and Control of Disease.* (1931)

Weger, George S. *The Liver in Fasting and Feasting.* (N.D.)

Wynn, Rev. Walter. *How I Cured Myself by Fasting.* (1925)

CASES OF FASTING

9 781428 626843

CPSIA information can be obtained
at www.ICGtesting.com
Printed in the USA
BVHW041958150720
583823BV00004B/472